"We have known Lyndon for There are unique qualities he make him stand out from the crowd. Among these are his inner strength, his ability to enthuse people around him and make them feel special. He is a natural encourager, a gifted motivator, a leader. There is never a dull moment around Lyndon because his sense of humour is infectious. He belongs to that special group of people who do what they say they are going to do. It is clear that his words are his bond and he definitely lives by them. We can count our friends on five fingers and many will be left out. But I have that certitude that Lyndon is a counted one, a true friend, somebody to laugh with, cry with and prepare to go to war with if needs be."

Martin and Noelie, Opticians, FBDO

"Lyndon oozes passion, whether it's cooking an omelette or analysing a business deal. He's a man who inspires other people to focus on a win-win solution. Lyndon never gives up. I've never known a guy to be constantly smiling...on the inside!"

Paul Evans, Retail and Business Director, Aurora Lighting

"Lyndon for the last three decades has engrossed himself within a world of positivity. This is a mental programming acquired by reading the correct books, listening to audios, watching videos, attending select seminars and associating with like-minded individuals. He understands that success, albeit mostly linked to financial success, is a mindset that all successful people acquire and it can be used in all areas of life. He has studied the footballers, baseball stars, athletes, business moguls, entrepreneurs and general TV personalities and found many common traits. Many of which he has fully adopted and if you have known Lyndon as long as we have, you will realise that he is passionate - he always is cheerful and encouraging - and more importantly always has that big smile!

We are startled to realise that he had used his positive mental attitude and skills to develop a routine/habit to treat his diabetes. Absolutely no way, in fact to him it would be the most natural path to follow. Lyndon has an amazing zest for life that is totally infectious and if you meet him personally, you will feel better for doing so!"

Roger and Paula Galloway,
Consultants for The Will Associates Ltd

"For a person to be able to achieve an extraordinary result in a short period of time, it comes down to a mindshift or a mindset. We believe the main reason why Lyndon Wissart has achieved this astonishing result involves a combination of self-esteem, father and husband responsibility, proudness and determination. Lyndon made the decision that enough was enough, he made the decision to take action so he can like what he sees in the mirror, not determined by outside circumstances. He made the decision to control what he eats, does and does not do. We believe Lyndon has achieved this extraordinary result because of his unique mindset and determination; combining both is a deadly weapon for success."

Richard and Maimuna Icare,
Icare Consulting Services

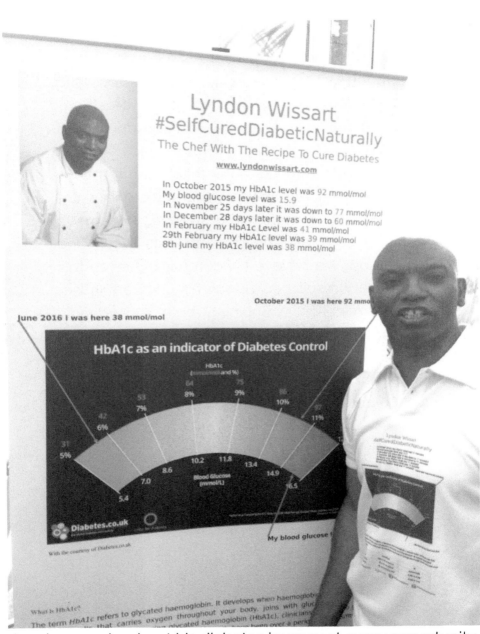

Lyndon speaks about his diabetes journey at every opportunity to help other people understand what they can achieve too.

About Lyndon

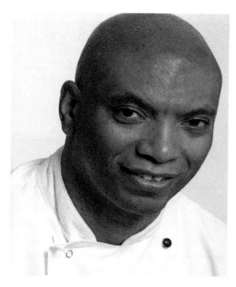

Hi, I am a professional British chef with more than 30 years' experience in all types of establishments, tasting and eating of all types of food. At the top of my list is desserts; this is my weakness.

I am passionate about creating amazing flavours and managing brilliant kitchens that provide the best customer experience possible. In October 2015, I was diagnosed with type 2 diabetes. I was not shocked, just a little surprised, because my cousin has had type 1 diabetes. I knew the symptoms and recognised several of them in myself.

But the great news – that I want to share with you in this book – is that in only 105 days, I self-cured my diabetes, by having a focused mindset on recovery and establishing a dedication to healthy nutrition and regular exercise, and I believe that you can do it too. This was done without medication. In this book, I will share my journey: my story, how I did it and exactly what I did, with no sugar coating! I will even provide you with my 'Five Fast Track approach', which you can try for yourself.

My Recovery Journey 2015 - 2016:
No sugar coating!

Date	Levels	Results	Impact
October 2015	HbA1c Blood Glucose	92 mmol/mol 15.9	Serious type 2 diabetes
November 2015	HbA1c	77 mmol/mol	Bad type 2 diabetes
December 2015	HbA1c Blood Glucose	60 mmol/mol 11.9	Average type 2 diabetes
February 2016	HbA1c	41 mmol/mol	Average type 2 diabetes
End of February 2016	HbA1c	39 mmol/mol	Reversed and controlled!
June 2016	HbA1c	38 mmol/mol	Reversed and feeling amazing!
October 2016	HbA1c	36 mmol/mol	Cured!

I have worked in many high-profile hotels and restaurants throughout London, including: the Savoy Hotel; Hamleys Toy Store; Café Royale; the Mount Royal Hotel; as well as catering for major indoor and outdoor events including: Wimbledon Championships; FNC Catering; BBC Centre; Gardner Merchant Catering; Royal Festival Hall; Spielsinger & Abrahams in North London; Inner London Crown Court; Collett Dickenson & Pearce; Lloyds Bank International; Wembley Stadium; Shelburne Hospital in High Wycombe; the Reform Club London; Adams Park; Eurest Corporate, a part of the Compass Group; Heathrow Airport Ltd; and the Farnborough Air Show.

In a freelance capacity, I have also worked with: James Zimmer Caterers; Jason Millan; Carole Sobell; Neil Samuels Ambassador Catering; Skye Cooks; Last Supper Ltd; Zafferano; Absolute Taste; Favour Catering; Celia Clyne; Capital Cooking; and Crème de la Crème.

I live with my wife and youngest daughter, with my grown-up son and two daughters close by. I grew up in London and I love reading, playing tennis, travelling, films, music, football, cycling, skiing and playing the drums.

I can be contacted in the following ways and would love to receive your feedback about my book and how it helps your life.

 @lwissart lwissart lwissart lwissart

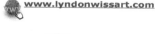 www.lyndonwissart.com

SEXY HIP MOVEMENTS

Lyndon the Dancing Chef!

AnnaMarie

Type 2 diabetes is not a life sentence,
it's an opportunity!

Lyndon Wissart

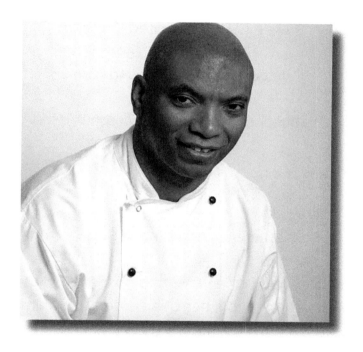

The Inspired Diabetic

How I cured my diabetes without medication

The chef with the recipe to cure type 2 diabetes

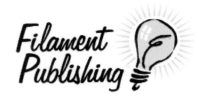

Published by Filament Publishing Ltd
16 Croydon Road, Beddington, Croydon,
Surrey, CR0 4PA, United Kingdom.
+44 (0)20 8688 2598
www.filamentpublishing.com

The Inspired Diabetic by Lyndon Wissart
© Lyndon Wissart 2017
ISBN 978-1-911425-18-2
Printed by IngramSpark

Illustrations by Anne-Marie Sonneveld

This book is not intended as a substitute for
the medical advice of physicians. The reader should
regularly consult a physician in matters relating
to his/her health and particularly with respect to
any symptoms that may require diagnosis
or medical attention.

Table of Contents

Dedications and Acknowledgements

My mum

I dedicate this book to my mother, Inez Adasa Wissart, who has been a rock in my life, loving and supporting me, giving me supportive advice and guidance. Her motto being; 'always get on with people' and this resonates every day in my life. Thank you, Mum.

My family

Yvonne, my wife; Jasmine, my daughter; and Babcia, my mother-in-law, who live with me and put up with my changing eating and exercising habits and supported me throughout this journey of recovery from type 2 diabetes. And, of course, my elder children, Shalena and my twins, Danielle and Leon.

My marketing, editing and publishing support team

Ken Williams, Richard Icare, Sherwyn Singh, Wendy Yorke, Anne-Marie Sonneveld, Chris Day and Darren St Mart, for what they have each done to support, guide and help me achieve my first book writing and publishing goal. I could not have done this without any of them.

Lyndon's Selected Type 2 Diabetes Dictionary: useful words for you to understand

Medical Terminology	Definition
Pancreas	The organ that produces insulin in your body
Insulin	The hormone that helps glucose to enter our cells and be used for energy
Beta Cells	The cells in the pancreas which produce insulin
Glucose	A commonly called sugar, which is an important energy source needed by all the cells and organs of our bodies. It comes from the digestion of carbohydrate and is also made by the liver
HbA1c	A measure of average blood glucose levels during 12 weeks (3 months)
Hyperglycaemia	High blood glucose
Hypoglycaemia	Low blood glucose
Impaired Glucose Tolerance (IGT) and Impaired Fasting Glycaemia (IFG)	States in which blood glucose levels are higher than normal, but not high enough to diagnose diabetes. People with IGT and IFG have an increased risk of cardiovascular disease and may go on to develop type 2 diabetes
Insulin Resistance	When the body is unable to make use of the insulin, it produces and glucose stays in the blood rather than moving into the body's cells for energy

Retinopathy	Caused when blood vessels in the eyes become blocked or leaky, and can damage vision if untreated
Neuropathy	Damage to the nerves, weakening their ability to transmit signals
Cardiovascular Disease	Diseases of the heart and circulation
IDD	Insulin-Dependent Diabetes
NIDD	Non-Insulin-Dependent Diabetes

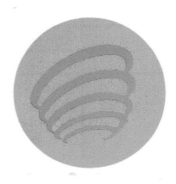

How this book can help you

Lyndon Wissart's journey of recovery explains what he did to turn his diabetes around, when he realised he was suffering the common symptoms of type 2 diabetes, including the following:

- always thirsty (*Polydipsia* is the medical term for excessive thirst, usually accompanied by a temporary or prolonged dryness of the mouth);
- frequently urinating (*Polyuria*);
- excessively hungry for no reason (*Polyphagia*);
- always tired;
- unexplained weight loss;
- genital itching;
- blurred vision;
- slow healing of cuts and bruising; and
- numbness in your hands and feet (pins and needles).

Why does Diabetes Create these Symptoms?

Lyndon's research taught him that these symptoms occur because some or all of the glucose in your blood, which is sugar, stays in the blood and is not being used as fuel for energy. The body tries to reduce blood glucose levels by flushing the excess glucose out of the body in the urine.

Lyndon discovered that the three main symptoms of diabetes are:

- *Hyperplasia* – unexplained increase in hunger, sometimes as a result of depression or stress;
- *Polydipsia* - increased thirst; and
- *Polyuria* - frequent, excessive urination.

> "The International Diabetes Federation estimates that between 80,000 and 100,000 children, representing some 50 countries, do not have consistent access to insulin"
>
> Provided by Beyond Type 1 Insulin for life
>
> @beyondtype1daily

Introduction:

Weight Gain and Weight Loss

Mindset

"Most people spend time documenting their talent instead of developing them, most people believe that talent creates success without effort. In a growth mindset, people believe their most basic abilities can be developed through dedication and hard work - brains and talent are just the starting point. This view creates a love of learning and a resilience that is essential for great accomplishment. Virtually all great people have had these qualities."

Carol Dweck

DIABETES
AROUND THE WORLD

8.3 PERCENT

% of US population with diabetes
25.8 million people
7th leading cause of death

285 MILLION

affected by diabetes world-wide
6.6% of total population
5th leading cause of death

COUNTRIES WITH THE LARGEST NUMBER OF PEOPLE WITH DIABETES

China
43.2 million

India
40.9 million

United States
25.8 million

Russia
9.6 million

Brazil
6 million

COUNTRIES WITH THE HIGEST PREVALENCE OF ADULT DIABETES

Nauru
30% diabetic

Bahrain
25.5% diabetic

United Arab Emirates
25% diabetic

Saudi Arabia
23.7% diabetic

Mauritius
20% diabetic

[The blue circle is the universal symbol for diabetes.]

Provided by Dr Bloem, Zurich, Switzerland

Since I can remember, I have been through the motions of eating healthily and thinking about exercising. But my weight was comfortable for me. I saw my older brother, Leslie, who was an avid exerciser and at times I wished I had the motivation like him to go running, play badminton and swim. But it was not there in me as it was in him.

I couldn't even swim. I had the confidence and the motivation to try with a fear of the water because of nearly drowning as a child. I had the powerful experience at a young age of seeing my life flash before me, as I had seen so many times in films or on TV, when someone is going down fighting the water, trying to climb to the top, but they keep on going down. To this day, I am grateful to the two guys who saved my life. We were on a school trip to Austria and this incident took place in a lake, when I was pushed into the water from a pier with all my clothes on. I was only 14 years old and I could not swim!

I also remember, when I was growing up I had individual swimming classes doing different exercises to see if I could float. My best memory is doing the mushroom exercise. This is when in the water you grab both legs at the ankles with both hands to form your body into a ball shape and in theory you should float to the top of the water. But, of course, I just went straight down to the bottom.

My brother was tall and slim with a flat stomach and I heard him on occasions make a sly remark about me, saying, 'Lyndon, your stomach is getting bigger.' But he didn't have to tell me, because I knew! I just did not do anything about it nor feel I needed to!

TYPE 2 DIABETES

DIABETES STATS

25.8 million
More than 8 percent of the U.S. population has been diagnosed with diabetes.

79 million
Approximately 35 percent of adults, 20 and older, have prediabetes — most have not been diagnosed.

71,382
The number of deaths directly attributed to diabetes annually in the United States. Diabetes also contributes to another 231,404 deaths per year.

2050
The year by which 1 in 3 Americans will have diabetes.

Types of Diabetes

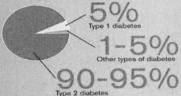

5% Type 1 diabetes

1-5% Other types of diabetes

90-95% Type 2 diabetes

Source: American Diabetes Association

PARTS OF THE BODY COMMONLY AFFECTED BY TYPE 2 DIABETES

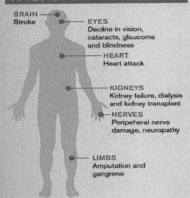

BRAIN Stroke

EYES Decline in vision, cataracts, glaucoma and blindness

HEART Heart attack

KIDNEYS Kidney failure, dialysis and kidney transplant

NERVES Peripeheral nerve damage, neuropathy

LIMBS Amputation and gangrene

HOW THE BODY REGULATES BLOOD GLUCOSE

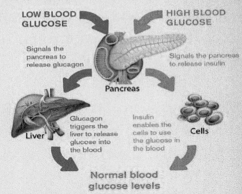

LOW BLOOD GLUCOSE
Signals the pancreas to release glucagon

HIGH BLOOD GLUCOSE
Signals the pancreas to release insulin

Pancreas

Glucagon triggers the liver to release glucose into the blood

Liver

Insulin enables the cells to use the glucose in the blood

Cells

Normal blood glucose levels

HOW THE BODY ATTEMPTS TO REGULATE HIGH BLOOD GLUCOSE IN TYPE 2 DIABETES

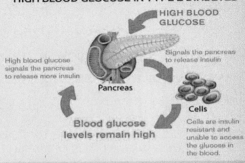

HIGH BLOOD GLUCOSE
Signals the pancreas to release insulin

High blood glucose signals the pancreas to release more insulin

Pancreas

Blood glucose levels remain high

Cells
Cells are insulin resistant and unable to access the glucose in the blood.

KNOW YOUR NUMBERS

Target Blood Glucose (mg/dl)

Fasting	Nonfasting (~2 hrs after a meal)
70-120	< 180

Hemaglobin A1c (%)

Normal	Prediabetes	Diabetes
<5.7	5.8-6.5	>6.5

Source: National Institute of Diabetes and Digestive and Kidney Diseases

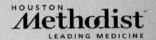

The day that something in me shifted and I knew I was getting bigger was when my mother, who was in her eighties by this point, said the same thing. That was a punch in the stomach for me and it hurt because all my life my mother was always supportive, caring and inspirational, motivating me to do good things. But she also spoke her mind openly.

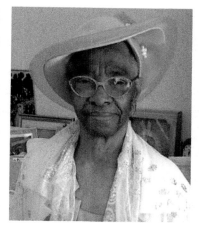

I remember looking in the mirror at myself and seeing that my face was chubby and round and my stomach was sticking out, although I could - just - see my toes! But my bum was large and I was wearing size 38 inch, 31 length, regular trousers, when I should have been wearing 36 inch. I was compensating for the large bum!

Being diagnosed with type 2 diabetes in October 2015 was a good and bad experience, depending how you see my situation. What it did for me was kick in the motivation that had always been there, but had never mentally connected when it came to food. In my mind, I knew what I was doing because I was a professional chef. But my diagnosis completely changed everything in my mind and I suddenly knew what I had to do and I was going to do it. I knew I had to lose weight and I had to lose my fatty stomach. I simply set my mental focus, my mindset, on reversing my diabetes. I started eating healthy foods and fitting in a regular, daily exercise routine, four times per week up to two hours per session in the gym.

I also started checking my weight every day and this kept me on track as a daily health check indicator and routine. Here is my weight loss table for that period of my life, which shows how

Weight Record Table 2015 – 2016

Date	Kilo	Stone	Comment
Sept/Oct	85/86	13.5	Fluctuating and rising!
November	84.5	13.5	Losing
December	83.4	13	Losing
18 December	81	12.7	Losing
23 December	79	12.5	Losing
13 January	80	12.6	In the morning
13 January	79.9	12.5	In the evening
15 January	81	12.7	Risen!
1 February	81	12.7	Stabilising?
5 March	77.6	12.2	Losing again
30 March	78.5	12.3	Stable
20 April	77	12.1	Losing
22 May	76.5	12	Looking good!
31 May	76	12	Happy
8 June	75.8	12	Feeling good
July	75	12	Feeling great!
August	75	12	Stabilised and Happy

quickly I was able to make it happen by putting my mind to it and staying focused on the goal. My determined mindset kicked in and I was suddenly motivated in a way I had not been for many, many years.

I looked myself in the eyes and I said the following affirmations out loud, to set my mindset on what I wanted to do!

- **'You can do it'** – to the subconscious mind
- **'I can do it'** – to the present existence
- **'I will cure my diabetes'**
- **'I will reverse my diabetes'**
- **'I will control my diabetes'**
- **'I have the ability'**
- **'This is a short-term process'**
- **'I will do what it takes'**
- **'I believe in me'**
- **'I am cured of being a diabetic'**

Motivation

During this period of weight loss, I received many positive and complimentary comments because I lost a total of 1.5 stone (about 10kg). Some people said it was not much when they saw me, but to me it was massive. And I remember the moment when I actually understood this and felt deeply good about it as a happy and significant moment in my recovery.

It was when I went to visit a friend, Jacques, who I had not seen for a few months. He ran a restaurant called The White Fish in Hendon, London and as I walked into his restaurant, I saw his wife, Ronni. She looked at me and said, 'Can I help you? What food would you like to order?' and looked down again at her cash register.

I called her name and she looked up again, but with a surprised look because she was confused and did not know how I knew her name. But as she looked up, she looked into my eyes and made a squelched, high-pitch noise and said, 'Lyndon, is that really you?' The look in her eyes, the expression on her face was amazing. Total shock and disbelief in how different I looked. She vigorously apologised, it was such a funny moment and we embraced each other.

The amount of compliments I have received has been outstanding. I had two friends who told me not to lose any more weight. Normal, healthy blood glucose levels, measured as the HbA1c level, are below 42mmol/mol. When my HbA1c went down to 41mmol/mol, I had achieved my ultimate goal. So what was there to do after that? I was feeling good, strong and energetic and above all, I was feeling healthy! In fact, I was feeling ecstatic, emotional and with tears of joy in my eyes.

Moderation

Once I had achieved my weight lose and my blood glucose level was back to a normal, non-diabetic level, I began to think about experimenting with my body by returning to eating the foods I had stopped eating, but in moderation. It was very rewarding to have small portions of my favourite food and feel good about it. My chef's interest in food kicked back in and I started to reintroduce flavours and colours again slowly and in smaller portion than I had been eating during my recovery period.

However, it is interesting that I drank none of my favourite fizzy drinks and fruit juices after my recovery, because I still did not have the desire for them.

I continued drinking water every day instead because it felt good. I did go back to drinking tea with milk, but with only one teaspoon of demerara sugar, which is something I am still adapting to, even now. Fortunately, my hot drink now is mainly peppermint tea, with lemon and ginger tea sometimes as well, with nothing else added, only hot water. I am happy I have found the drink I enjoy. This is important for me and demonstrates I have developed new tastes and have discovered more food choices now than I have ever had before. This has been a significant, but unexpected outcome of my diabetes journey from 2015 – 2016 and why I want to share my story to help you have the same positive and healthy result, if that is what you want too.

After going back to eating my normal food, I continued to lose weight from February to March 2016 and the most amazing thing was that, on 29 February, my HbA1c level went down to 39mmol/mol. I was not going to the gym as often as before nor doing a full workout. The only thing I can put this down to is the fact that I was having my cayenne pepper drink with fresh lemon juice and at times with spirulina, cloves and cinnamon. Or I was having my okra water as my basic drink every day, which must have aided me losing more weight.

The good news was I had lost my fatty stomach and I could see the lines of my teenage six-pack showing up again! My face looked slimmer, my large bum had disappeared. To celebrate, I decided to treat myself to a new pair of trousers in a size 36 inch regular. But they did not fit me properly because they were too long and I had to get 36 short 29 length. 'I must have shrunk,' I thought to myself!

There was another occasion when I was going out after work but I forgot to pack my trousers. So in a rush, I had to buy a new pair. At the shop, I went for the 36 inch short range and they looked and felt really good, if a little baggy. I had to buy a belt to keep the trousers up. I was in a hurry and did not want to waste time because I was meeting someone who had travelled some distance to see me. When I arrived, the first thing they commented on was how my trousers looked a bit baggy but I did not think much about it.

However, when I got home, I asked my trusted wife what she thought about the new trousers and with her open honesty, she said they looked too big and didn't fit me properly. So I took the belt off and the trousers simply fell off! They were too big at 36 inch, I could have fitted into a 34 inch short trouser after all and I was certainly shrinking but I was also so happy to have achieved my goal and turned my diabetes around!

It is hard to explain the deep sense of satisfaction I felt and that is why I am sharing my story of how I did it.

By reading this book, you are taking the first step, just as I did back in 2015 when I was first diagnosed.

Congratulations!

PART ONE:
MINDSET

"The first step
toward success is taken
when you refuse to be a captive of
the environment in which
you first find yourself."

Mark Caine

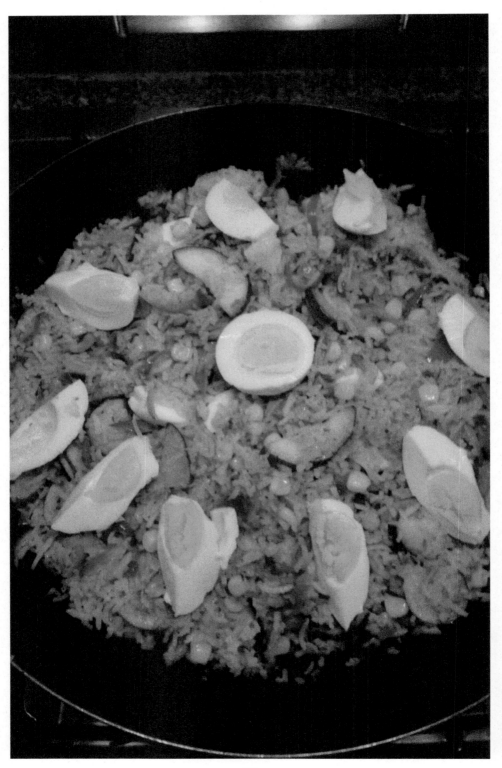

Chapter 1

Pre-diagnosis: sweet innocence

I have a good friend who lives in Poland named Bogdan Wojcik and I went to stay with him once a year. I always found this very refreshing, after working hard in a hot kitchen for the rest of the year, and I always came back full of renewed energy and motivation.

In January 2014, I went to a honey-processing factory in Poland with Bogdan, where they mentioned the natural benefits of honey keeping the common cold away. Of course, they recommended local organic honey, but I found it expensive and not easy to get hold of at the time, so when I returned home I chose to buy normal honey off the supermarket shelf. I liked honey and I started having it in my tea and coffee and everything else possible as well! In my coffee, I added a teaspoon as well as the two teaspoons of brown sugar I had put in my drink already.

However, it got to the stage where I was running out of honey so quickly because I was buying 350g small bottles one at a time and using it in so many foods - I was defiantly trying to keep the flu away! No colds, no flu, no medication, no extra vitamin tablets and I felt great, but it was a disastrous habit to let myself fall into.

As a chef, I had access to shop in a Cash and Carry warehouse and I bought packs of honey in bulk, as well as latte coffee sachets, full of sugar already. To these coffee sachets, I added milk or water and the way I liked it best was to add one third hot water and the rest hot milk with two teaspoons of additional brown sugar. I also added a teaspoon of honey - to keep the bugs away!

As I walked around the Cash and Carry warehouse, I saw all my sweet weaknesses, for example, digestive biscuits with milk chocolate and childhood sweets. I wanted to have a healthy breakfast on the cold winter mornings and I thought, 'What better way to start the day than to have porridge oats.' I brought the normal oats in the box, and after boiling them forever, they burnt in the pan! However, with a sprinkle of brown sugar, a squirt of honey and the occasional double cream for that extra full body flavour and smooth texture, they were a treat for breakfast! I changed from using refined white sugar to brown demerara sugar because I was told it was healthier. My wife introduced me to two-minutes-in-the-microwave-porridge, which I had my doubts about, until I discovered the oats are no different except they are cooked for longer. I decided to go for the golden syrup two-minute porridge oat sachet, but the trouble was, I added a squirt of my favourite honey and a sprinkle of demerara sugar to the already sweetened porridge.

Also, I wanted to add a bit more of a healthier option into the porridge with more flavour and I added sultanas and raisins, which of course were delightfully sweet and added more colour and texture. At the warehouse, I bought 5kg demerara sugar packs to save me money, rather than the 5 x 250g bags. I had not realised they sold the chocolate pallets we used in the restaurant kitchens. These would be great for me to have at home, 2.5kg bags of dark, milk and white chocolate. They were easy to melt to make muffins and most importantly for me to snack on! Especially when the computer cupboard was next to the food cupboard in our house where the chocolate was meant to be safe!

On one occasion at the warehouse, on a big yellow board they were advertising a discount of J2o cherry flavour juice drinks. I was keen to try a new flavour because the mango and passion fruit or orange I was already drinking always gave me heartburn. I thought I cannot go wrong with the cherry juice, so I bought 2 x 24 bottle cases. What a relief to taste something different. Two bottles of the new juice went straight into the fridge when I arrived home and I could not wait to have a cool refreshing drink, full of flavour, with my evening meal. And what a treat that was, but of course I went for another one and then quickly had to go to the bathroom to pee it out! It was a different flavour, but it had a similar effect as the other flavoured drinks and gave me heartburn but I took no notice of these irritating impacts and did not know at the time that they were pre-diabetic symptoms, I simply focused on the flavour! Or was I in denial? With 24 bottles of J2o in the house waiting for me to indulge, that is exactly what I did daily. For some reason, I was peeing more often, but I thought it was normal, because I was drinking more liquid.

What I did not realise, was that I was learning to live with the symptoms of diabetes without knowing it. This was a big mistake and I hope by reading my book, you will not take the same path. Instead, seek help and change what is going on in your life immediately you become aware of these changes. They are signals from your body telling you to take actions, rather than ignoring them!

I was aware I needed to lose weight and my good friend Sherwyn Singh advised me to drink natural prune juice. He said it would help me to lose weight quickly as a laxative, helping me to go to the toilet more! But of course, it was also full of sugar and I was drinking it every other day and thinking it was helping my diet – how sweetly innocent was I at that stage, or was I in denial about my health and my weight? As a chef, I knew these nutritional facts, but I was not applying them to my body, only to my daily work in the restaurant kitchens!

At this time, I was working in a kitchen on the pastry section where every morning we had to prepare cakes. We trimmed the edges and cut the cakes into portions. Of course, I used to think, 'Why waste the edges and throw them away, when I can eat them later or with my morning latte with sugar and honey? Why not top up on my energy level first thing on a cold winter morning?' At times, when there was an excess of cake trimmings, we gave some to the other chefs.

It was coming up to rugby world cup season and it was exciting because as a self-employed chef, this meant regular work for me and a few weeks' stint work would be good for my pocket. We were preparing a lot of food for the rugby world cup and there were lots of dessert tastings, a chef's delight. Many chefs came into the pastry section and asked for the leftovers or if there was anything sweet they can have, but as the pastry chefs we had the pleasure of first choice! Of course, there was very little left for those disappointed chefs when I was there!

As the rugby world cup got underway, it was getting busier and busier and I had to leave home at 5:30am to beat the traffic and also to get a parking space at work. My routine then was to make a flask of tea including my usual sugar and honey and, together with three slices of granary bread spread with jam, take these with me for my one-hour car journey! And this was before I had my breakfast and started working, but at the time I did not think about what I was doing to my body!

My evening meals were a variation of 'what you see is what you eat'. My wife is not an avid cook but when she wants to, she can really cook a good meal. However, this was less frequent because she is a professional, usually leaving home early in the morning and returning home late at night. Because my mother-in-law lives with us and is Polish, it was hard sometimes to know if what she had cooked something we would like. She was diagnosed with breast cancer a few years ago and had changed her eating habits to include the types of food we were not accustomed to eating. At times when she cooked, we had the choice to join her or not.

As I was not sure if there was food at home in the evening or whether it would be anything I liked, I was in the habit of buying takeaway on my way home. Burger meals were one of my favourites and also pulled chicken. I also called the local Chinese takeaway en route home and place my order to be ready for me and not to waste too much time waiting for the meal. I went through a phase of having large spring rolls (delicious!) until one day a spring roll only had bean sprouts inside and a couple of peas and I could not tell what else was in there (and I'm a chef) so that ended. Often, I went to my local Caribbean takeaway, especially with my daughter, and there was no holding back on choices. My favourite was stewed chicken rice and peas with plantain, and my daughter loved the curried goat. My sneaky snack was the Jamaican patty, in any flavour.

When I was at home, I usually cooked for the family, depending on each person's personal taste or requests, especially my daughter, Jasmine. I cooked fish dishes or meat - predominantly chicken; stir-fry meat and vegetables; stir-fry rice; pasta with cheese sauce (Jasmine's favourite) - and I used to add bacon and chicken to make it really delicious. On Sundays, I cooked fully-loaded roast chicken or lamb with all the trimmings. I love my food and so does my family!

When my wife and I were busy working, we depended more on my mother-in-law, who is an awesome cook. With her being at home, there was always some cooked food. She cooked a variety of meals, including soups, which was a regular occurrence. Some of her favourite soups included: tomato soup with rice and cream; fresh vegetable soup; and courgette soup with Dolcelatte cheese. There was a routine of the same foods, including beef lasagne, which we all liked, as well as Polish dishes, including: pierogi: kielbasa polish meats: bigos (sauerkraut stew with pork): zurek Polish soup: golabki - pronounced gawampki (mincemeat wrapped white cabbage): and schabowi (pork chop flattened and coated in egg and breadcrumbs and shallow fried).

There were times I enjoyed a fry-up with fried eggs, baked beans, bacon or sausages, chips, cod in batter, which I loved dearly - the crispy batter surrounding fresh cod!

We have a family joke. When my wife says there is nothing to eat because she did not look in the fridge, I go through the fridge and see what foods I find and create something out of nothing. As a chef, I can get creative, but my wife says she is not hungry. However, when she smells what I am cooking, she comes to the kitchen and says, 'That looks and smells great.' I tease her by dishing up one plate of food and eating it in front of her. When she asks where is hers, I politely remind her she is not hungry - before getting her some.

After a meal there was usually a desire for more: a dessert, ice cream or something sweet like cakes or digestive chocolate biscuits. Not good for us but we all enjoyed them!

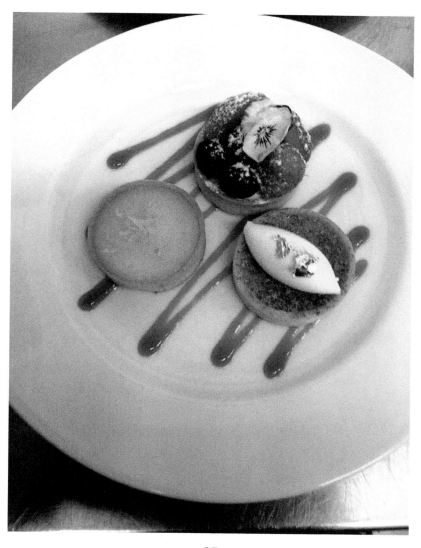

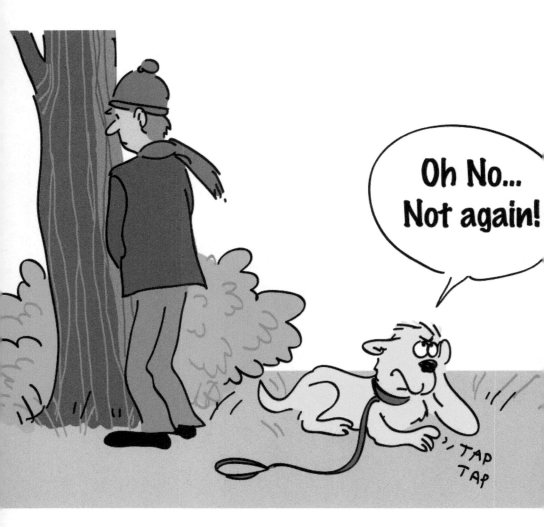

Symptom: Frequent Urination

Chapter 2

Symptoms:
Jelly Baby addiction!

I was getting incredibly busy at work, cutting cakes, eating the cake trimmings with my coffee and enjoying my oats porridge for breakfast almost every day. This habit was making me thirstier and I drank more and more water without realising what was happening to my body. I started to go for a pee more often.

At work, we were not allowed to use the toilets in the main building where we worked. We had to go to another building about 50 metres further away. At first it was OK. When I felt I wanted to go to the toilet, I went in a relaxed fashion, but as time progressed, when I thought I could hold it, the urge became more sudden and I had to step up my pace to get to the toilet in time. This habit became increasingly urgent and it got to the stage where the staff toilet was too far away to walk to and I had to sprint to the nearest toilet, which was the one we were not allowed to use! But I did not care because unless I did this, I was in trouble and unable to hold it anymore! As soon as I felt it, I knew I had to go.

Another problem I learnt to live with, was an odd feeling when I was at work standing in the kitchen or at home, as if something was beside me. When I turned to look, there was nothing there,

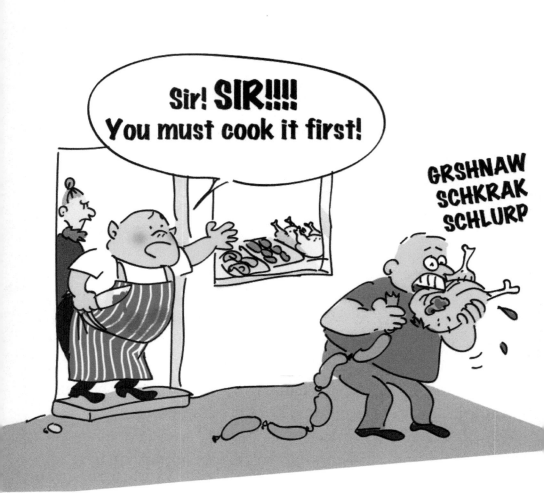

Symptom: Excessive Hunger

but I noticed my eyes were blurred and my focusing a bit fuzzy! I rubbed my eyes and they watered for no reason. Or I was reading a recipe at work with my glasses on and there was sometimes a blur I could not explain!

I was also constantly tired, but I couldn't understand why because I had so much sugar in my system and I should have been full of energy! When I was at home or out driving and feeling tired, I would naturally reach for a snack bar or a packet of Jelly Babies, which I always made sure I had plenty of in my car and at home, to give me that extra bit of energy, or so I thought! I was working in London but travelling to Ramsgate regularly to visit family and so I drove my car to work. I always had two bags of 1kg Jelly Babies to eat on the journey to keep me awake and alert as I was driving. I ate a sweet when I felt like I needed one, which was constantly. I also always had two sugars in my tea and I loved my fizzy drinks. I went through stages of drinking only Fanta and sometimes Pepsi. When I got tired of drinking Coca Cola, my luxury drink was Ginger Beer.

I noticed I was often hungry straight after eating a meal and I wanted to eat again! I also had a skin disorder where my skin became whiter and whiter. I didn't think much of this because I knew it was called a snow process and I had heard of it before! Occasionally, I showed my friends during a close conversation when we had a heart to heart. I revealed my chest area, where the different shade of brown to white or lighter brown skin was more obvious, but neither they nor I thought much about what it might mean.

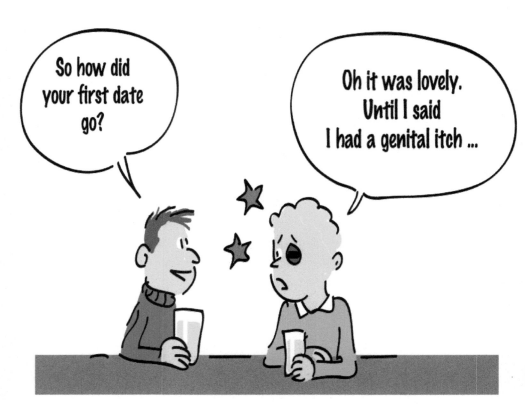

Symptom: Genital Itch

At the same time these symptoms were creeping up on me, I was slowly gaining more and more weight. I was aware of it and thinking I needed to do something about it, but I did nothing differently. There seemed no point in worrying, no motivation either! I was drinking so much water but it had became a pleasure to drink water which I thought was healthy. I always had at least one or two bottles of water in my car and when I was travelling I constantly drank water. It simply became a good habit for me.

While I was experiencing these symptoms and the slow weight gain, I was happy in my life and I was in a good environment doing what I do best, working as a chef as I had done for many years.

About this time, I noticed blood in my stool, but there was no pain going to the toilet or soreness, so I thought there was nothing to worry about. However, I experienced a reddish, itchy rash on my genitals. I had no idea why it was there and I asked myself, 'How could I have this? What is happening here?' I tried self-medication using antiseptic to smooth the pain and fight infection. This became a daily treatment to eradicate the itching, but the cure was not instant and the itching was continuous because it rubbed against my underwear. When it did ease off slowly, it was such a relief, but it was to return again.

I was still gaining weight slowly and always saying I needed to exercise while never doing it. I went through the phase with my wife of taking part in an exercise programme on YouTube but I was putting food into my mouth at the same time! Of course, I knew this was not how I should be behaving, but I was happy and life was good!

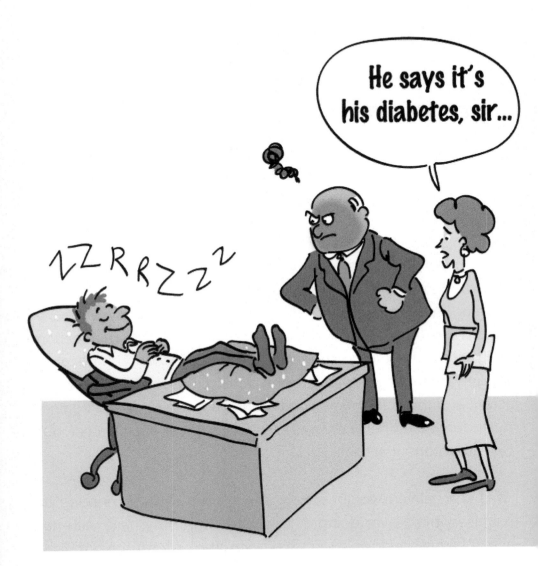

Symptom: Always Tired

I began to feel the effects on my body. As my stomach got larger, I weighed myself and thought I need to be exercising and to reduce the intake of certain food. I looked at recipe books for healthy food but being a chef, I said to myself, 'I know what I should be eating and what not to eat.'

Oh yeah, was I a chef in denial, knowing the facts but not making it happen for myself! I was certainly in denial about my state of health, looking for answers rather than acting on the questions. In our house, we have an electronic weighing scale in the bathroom on the floor on the left-hand side as you enter. You cannot miss it and it is a great reminder to use it (yeah right!) or to bypass it, which I did on many occasions.

My constant tiredness was becoming worse and more noticeable. I went to bed earlier or I fell asleep on the sofa watching TV with the side lamp on. I was having a good eight hours of sleep, waking up and having a shower and breakfast, but then feeling as if I could go back to bed and sleep again! I actually did this on some occasions when I was not working and no one else was in the house! I was mentally motivated to get up and go, but my body was reluctant to follow or join the motivation.

I remember my wife saying, 'Lyndon, come to bed,' while I was dosing off in front of the TV or the computer. I thought she was nagging me, but I was mistaken. She saw I was not myself, not the normal smiling, caring, motivated, get it done now person who Lyndon was.

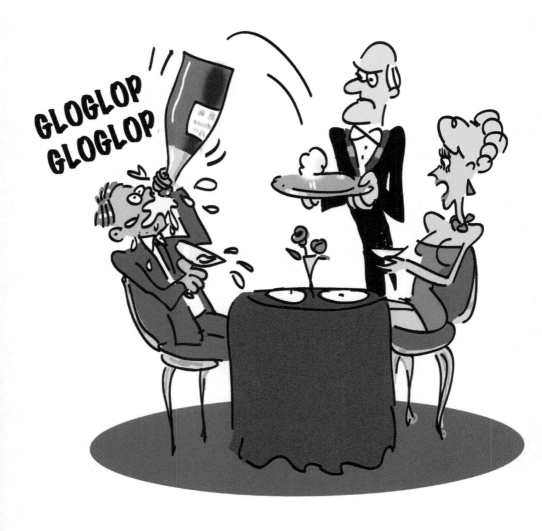

Symptom: Always Thirsty

Also, as mentioned, I was visiting the toilet more often than usual; was it because I was drinking more and more and I was always thirsty, needing something to drink? When working in a kitchen, it was a courtesy to let the head chef you were working with know you were going to the toilet, to let them know you were not skiving or going for a quick cigarette break. I felt myself informing the chef more and more often, to the point when I became self-conscious about asking again.

Also, I remember, on separate occasions and at different times, people I was working with told me how red my eyes were looking and how tired I looked in my face, but I was fine, I felt OK and took no notice!

Sometimes when I was sitting on the toilet, I noticed tingles in my feet. It was a strange feeling that brought back memories of when I was skiing and wearing heavy and uncomfortable ski boots. My feet used to sting with pins and needles and feel numb at the bottom. It was a very uncomfortable experience and I remembered how nice it used to be and such a relief to loosen or even take off my boots at lunchtime when we stopped skiing for a break and what a relief it was to have no pain.

I noticed, while sitting on the toilet and being reflective for a moment having a break from work, that on occasions I had a slight pain on the lower, left-hand side of my stomach. I noticed this pain when sitting down, especially when driving. I put my hand there and gave it a poke or a rub to see if there was anything there, such as a lump. But as I pushed where the pain was, I found nothing and I kept telling myself it was simply an annoying, uncomfortable ache.

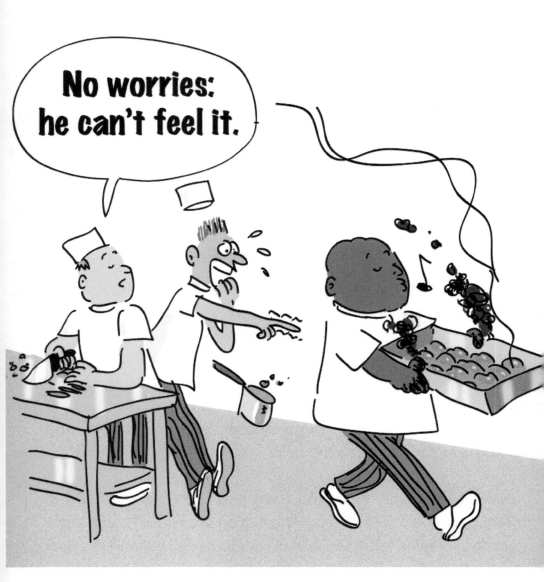

Symptom: Numbness

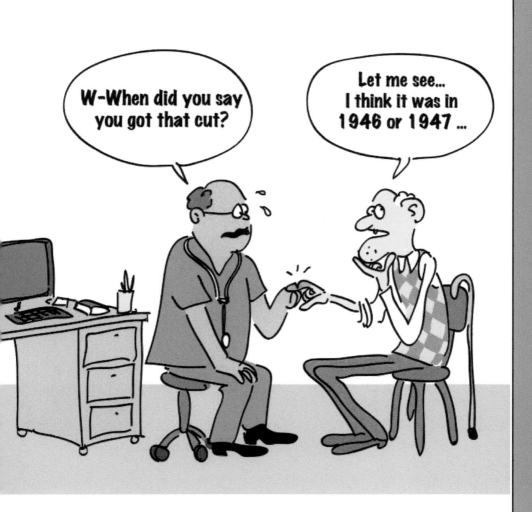

Symptom: Slow Healing

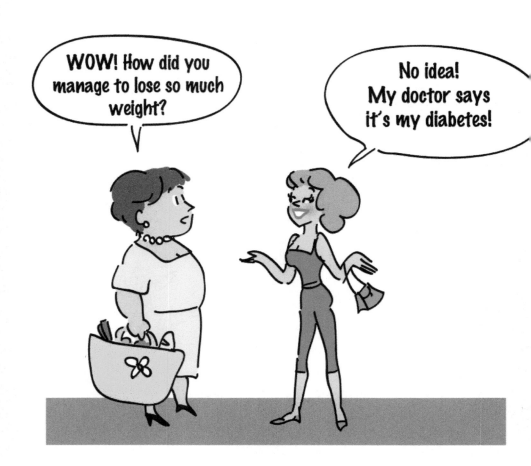

Symptom: Weight Loss

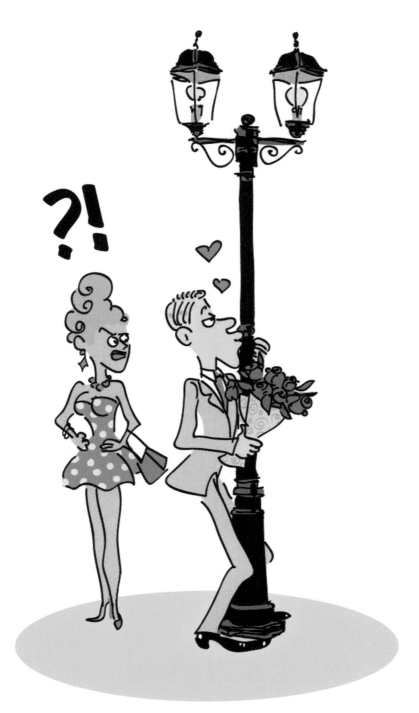

Symptom: Blurred Vision

Diet Change

Lyndon started by following the UK's National Health Service Steps to a Healthy Diabetic Diet, as provided below.

Eat regular meals	At least three a day
Cut down on sugar and sugary foods and drinks	Use diet, low-sugar or sugar-free squashes and fizzy drinks. Sugary drinks cause blood glucose levels to rise quickly
Eat more low-sugar fruit and cruciferous vegetables	Aim for at least five servings of fruit and vegetables a day. This will provide you with vitamins and fibre, and help make your diet more balanced
Cut down on the fat you eat and include more beans and pulses in your diet	Particularly animal fats because this type of fat is linked to heart disease. Eating less fat and fatty foods will also help you lose weight. Grill, steam or oven bake rather than frying foods
Use less salt	Use herbs and spices to flavour food rather than adding salt

If you drink alcohol, take in moderation	For women, two units a day For men, three units per day
	Never drink on an empty stomach because alcohol can increase the likelihood of hypoglycaemia (low blood sugar levels)

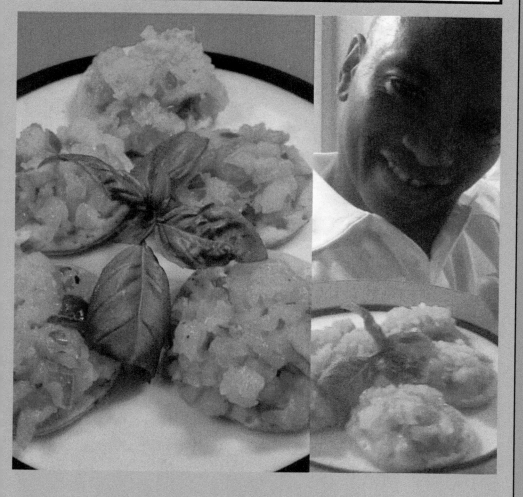

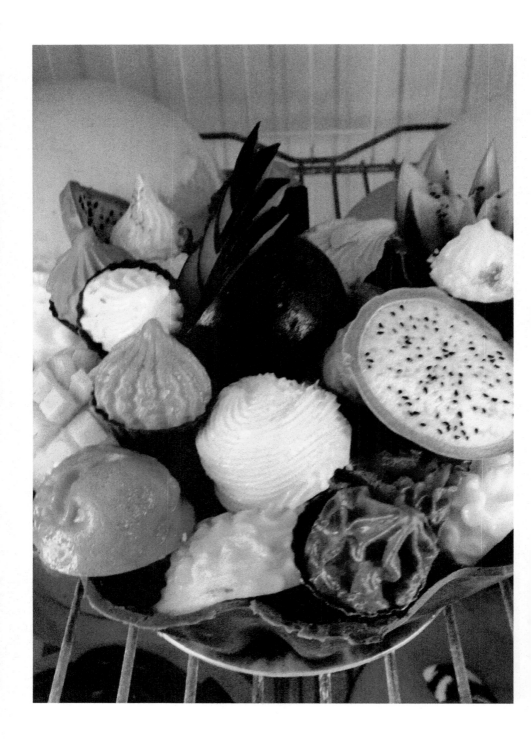

Chapter 3

Diagnosis:
from black to white

Eventually, I went to see my doctor on 16 October 2015 because of the now constant pain in my lower stomach. As I waited to see the doctor, I thought about what I was going to say, a man in denial about his health situation. The doctor asked me how she could help me and I explained the symptoms and problems I was experiencing, including the stomach pain and blood in my stool.

She asked me to lie down on the bench where she had rolled out the clean, white tissue paper. I lay on my back and showed her where the pain was in my stomach. However, she couldn't find anything abnormal after prodding it with her hands and fingers. She recommended I have a colonoscopy and flexible sigmoidoscopy procedure that she booked for me, and she took my blood pressure, which was normal. She gave me a blood glucose level test, which I had never had before, and it read 15.9. She said straight away that was not good: 'You will probably have diabetes.' I was not shocked as I was expecting something like this because of my symptoms. My cousin Ken had type 1 diabetes and I knew a little information about it from research I had done before. It was at that point, when the doctor told me my blood glucose level was not good, that I instantly said to myself, 'I am not having sugar anymore.' It was a black or white decision in my head, my heart and soul.

It simply came to me. I said to myself, 'That's enough; it is time to act, Lyndon, time to do something differently and change this now.'

The hospital procedure I was going to have was an investigation using a flexible tube to look accurately at the lining of the large bowel, up to the sigmoid colon. The long tube, called a colonoscope, is inserted up the anus and manoeuvred around the left-hand side of the bowel. It has an illumination channel which enables light to be directed onto the lining of the bowel and it relays pictures back onto a television screen. This facilitates the endoscopist to have a clear view and to check whether the bowel is normal.

There was a pre-preparation procedure, a low fibre diet, taken two days prior to starting the prescribed bowel cleansing medication. This was MoviPrep, a strong form of laxative. It was recommended not to drive after the procedure so my wife escorted me to the hospital. We went into the reception and found comfortable seating in the waiting area. We had a brief conversation, but I had a nervous tone to my voice and I was agitated because I was not used to being in a hospital for medical treatment.

When the nurse called my name, I went to her with my bag of items. She gave me a gown to change into which I did and sat down and waited with a book to read. When I was called up, I went into the room where there were four welcoming nurses, all with smiles of comfort. One nurse said to me, 'You have your gown the wrong way around,' and I made a joke about it. When that was corrected, I was asked to sit on the bed and there was a TV screen in front of me.

The four nurses approached me and I was nervous, holding back a tear, with my emotions thinking, 'What am I doing here? How did I let myself go so far to be in this position?' The nurses looked at me intently as one of them started to ask me questions.

How long and how regularly had I had blood in my stool? But the question that got me was: What colour was the blood, dark red, light red, and can you describe it? I replied it was light red and was surprised by the simultaneous smiles from all the nurses. 'That is good,' the nurse said. What a huge relief I felt. It meant it was fresh blood and not so serious. I was instructed to lie down on my side for the procedure to start. I saw the flexible sigmoidoscopy illuminating up my bowel and relaying the pictures back to the television screen.

After the procedure was finished, I thanked the nurses and they said goodbye with great humility and smiles. I went back to the waiting room, got changed and waited for the nurse. She came out and showed me that the results were all normal, except that I had small haemorrhoids, which was the cause of the blood in my stool. A bloody relief!

As all was normal from the flexible sigmoidoscopy, I was referred for an ultrasound scan at the NHS Diagnostic Centre. The examination was for an upper abdomen and urinary tract and it was due to take place on 8 December 2015. For the preparation, I had to fast for six hours prior to my appointment. I was only allowed to drink clear fluids, although the instructions I received said diabetics were allowed to eat two slices of dry toast with jam (no dairy products) but not within two hours of the appointment.

I was prepared and as I waited for my procedure, I was alone clutching my book looking at it trying to read, but my mind and my eyes were travelling somewhere else. Then 9.20am came and my name was not called yet. I had arrived 15 minutes early and sitting there felt like a long time, with other patients coming and going and me continuing to sit there.

I had no reception on my telephone and I went for a walk outside to check on my social network updates and to take my mind away from what was happening to me!

Finally, I was called and as I entered the room and saw the monitors, a bit of anticipation set in. As I lay down on the bench, the cold gel came across my abdomen and I looked at the screen and saw my body parts in black and white. The doctor was explaining what we were looking at and after he had finished, I wiped the gel off my abdomen and asked if everything was normal. He said one of my kidneys was in the wrong place and I had a fatty liver. The doctor mentioned that with exercise and diet, I can reduce the fat in the liver. There was nothing related to my abdominal pains with no abnormalities showing up on the scan. I was happy and relieved, although confused and unsure why I had this pain.

A few days after this, I went to visit a friend, Prosper Bitton, at his bakery, Crème de la Crème in Temple Fortune, Golders Green, London. I told him about my abdominal scan and that I had a fatty liver. He recommended I drink lemon water first thing in the morning. I took his advice and started drinking lemon water the next day and I continue to do this on a regular basis. I simply juice a lemon into water every day and drink it with nothing else added. It became a health ritual to help my fatty liver recover.

Prosper also recommended olive leaves tea. I had a Greek friend called Dina who I asked to send me some olive leaves. This was an alternative tea for me and although I did not like the taste, I knew my body needed the health benefits and it was worth drinking.

The doctor booked me for a blood test, for the blood glucose level HbA1c, on Monday 19 October 2015. At this point, I became more concerned because this blood test was to check that everything was alright. I asked the doctor to conduct all the tests at the same time to provide me with a complete health picture, and for this reason I kept the test to myself. I guess I did this because I knew it was not a good sign. I could not tell my wife, although I thought calling her on the telephone would be easier than to tell her to her face. I was wrong, because as soon as she answered the telephone, I could not control my emotions. With tears running down my cheeks, I told her we would talk later speaking in gibberish and with a trembling voice.

On Tuesday 20 October 2015, the day after my first blood test, I was working in the kitchen when my telephone rang. I didn't recognise the number, but it was my local area code so I answered. 'Hello, is this Mr Wissart? Your blood test shows us you are diabetic'. There was no compassion in her voice, it was just another telephone call to make and she got straight to the point. She said I would have to see a dietician and gave me a date and time for eight days later, with no more information and that was it. With only one day before my birthday, I remember thinking, 'What a great gift!'

When I finished the telephone call, the realisation began to kick in. There was no one around me I could dry my eyes on.

The first person I told was Ivan, a chef who worked with me. I simply shouted out to him across the kitchen, 'I have type 2 diabetes'. I don't even remember exactly how I said it. Except I remember that it sounded to me as if I was talking about someone else, not me! And to be honest, at that moment I didn't totally understand what it meant. Again, I was in denial. Another chef I worked with called Angela came into the kitchen and started to work at her station. My lips were trembling. How can I tell her? I looked at her and said, 'I have type 2 diabetes', as if it wasn't me I was talking about and I recall a strange 'out of body' feeling. She was very comforting and gave me words of encouragement, which I needed at the time and were welcomed.

I remember this moment in my life felt terrible. How could I be here? I shouldn't be here – mentally I knew the right things to do but I hadn't been doing them. For example, eating sweet foods and drinking too many fizzy drinks that I knew were not good for me and not taking regular exercise. I remember a feeling of failure and fear creeping in: Did this mean I couldn't work? Could I still earn a living and look after my family? I didn't know what effect this condition was going to have on my life and the life of the people around me – my nearest and dearest. At the same time, I was trying to stop myself from feeling these fears because I knew I was overreacting and much worse things happen to other people. This was only diabetes after all and type 2, not type 1, which would have been so much worse.

PART TWO:
MOTIVATION

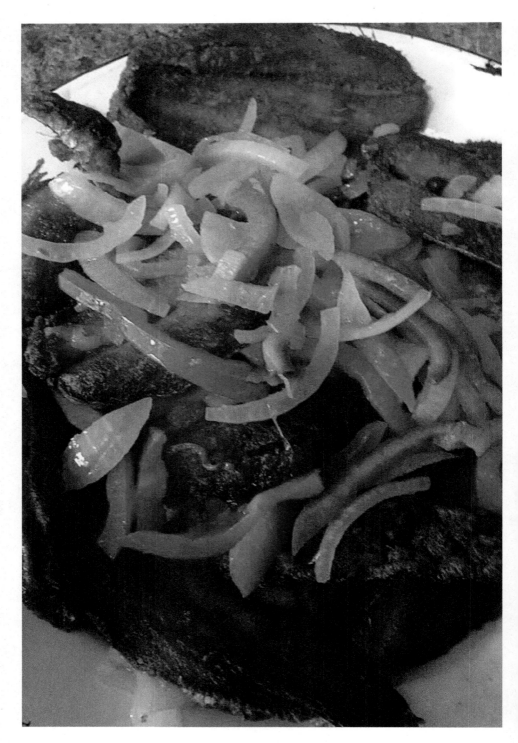

Lyndon's mother's fried fish

Chapter 4

Overcoming Reluctance: advice from family and friends

The day I received the diagnosis telephone call when I was at work, was a very slow day in the kitchen, but I had so much going on in my head everything felt as if it was going in reverse. I was regretting eating all those cake trimmings when I should have given or thrown them away. Images of all the things I had been doing wrong for my body, including: the coffee with two teaspoons of sugar topped up with honey; the extra sweets; luxury snacks; and instant porridge oats with golden syrup - my healthy option - yeah right! And all those fizzy drinks and sugary juices! These pictures were all going round and round in my head attacking me.

It was a difficult time, not being able to control my tears trickling down my face, an odd feeling on my cheeks I was not used to. I could not even say, 'Pull yourself together, Lyndon,' because I was together. I just needed to know what my next step was.

To be honest, my next step should have been to call my cousin Ken, who had type 1 diabetes, because when he eventually told me his story, I was blown away. Once I understood what he had been through, there were nights when I could not sleep.

Flashback One - my cousin Ken

A few months before I was diagnosed, I went to visit my cousin Ken. I wanted to discuss a business idea with him so we sat down in his front room. We were in a general chatty mood, although I was keen to talk about my business idea. But with his personality of fast forward speaking, he was quick to tell me what had happened to him. I hadn't seen Ken for quite some time, and it was a good time to catch up. I was excited about talking to him about my new business project but as I started to talk to him about it, I knew there was something he wanted to say to me. He was hesitant at first and then he told me what had happened to him when he was diagnosed with type 1 diabetes and he had been able to reverse it.

However, at that moment, before I knew about my situation, this didn't mean much to me. But he carried on telling me about how we got his diabetes. He said it was stress-related and it was so bad, he had been hospitalised and had been through a near-death experience. I couldn't believe that I had not known about it, considering we were close cousins and that he had not told me about this before and nobody in my family had informed me either!

He showed me his insulin and Metformin medication boxes. They were piled high and looked like a shelf in a chemist. He told me how he was taking the insulin daily via injections and I was shocked. He also showed me how he checked his blood glucose levels and the blood level monitor. The one thing I could not comprehend was when he took his blood test and put the reading into his computer to read it. This was a bit technical for me. I didn't understand it but I was fascinated to see how technology had come such a long way for testing blood in your home! He went on to tell me about the food he was eating and I was surprised to find out how basic and simple it was. Being a chef, I thought it sounded a bit bland with little flavour, texture or colour in his new diet. We had an extensive conversation that evening with Ken speaking about diabetes all the time and suddenly it was time for me to go home without discussing my business plan, which was left for another day.

I don't think he really wanted to discuss it in detail, but I understood, because of what he had been through during the last year. It had obviously been very traumatic and I thought I had to listen to him.

On the way home driving my car, my thoughts were racing back to what he had said. I saw all kinds of pictures in my head of what he was going through. It was like a whirlwind in my mind and I remember thinking, 'I don't know if I could put up with what he has been through.' His story was so intriguing that I could not sleep properly that night, it must have been a dream. For days, his story was playing on in my mind. I was thinking that he must tell his story, he must share it, write a book, produce a short video to tell other people about what he had achieved.

The next day, I called Ken and asked him if he had thought about writing a book detailing his story, to help other people around the world with the same problems. He said he had thought about it but not done it yet! 'Great,' I remember replying and I was relieved.

᪥

I was never around people with diabetes before but the only other time I can remember was when my friend Alan's mum was not well and I went to visit her at home. I went into the room where she was sitting with her legs up on a chair with a chequered blanket over her legs. I looked into her eyes and she looked at me and said (in a Jamaican strong patwa accent), 'Da sugar get mi it get mi bad'. I did not understand what she meant but she was referring to diabetes and that is how she said it. A few months later, she passed away. I never forgot that experience and now it came back to haunt me.

The following day, 21 October 2015, I was busy making a batch of 20 litre lemon curd. I was weighing out the ingredients when a colleague Tameka came up to me and said her granddad had type 2 diabetes. I looked at her as if to say, 'I don't remember telling you my problem.' I replied saying, 'I am sorry to hear that,' and carried on working. I was working at the hot stove, still adjusting to my situation. When you are making a batch of lemon curd, you need to continuously keep on stirring, to stop it sticking or burning. I was stirring with a whisk and feeling the red heat. Tameka came to me again and swiftly said, I don't mean to bother you, Lyndon' - her body language was not full on in front of me because she was to my side - so she could say what she wanted before she moved back to the table where she was working. But she was trying to be helpful, saying, 'Lyndon, my granddad has this product called spirulina, which he takes every day to help with his diabetes.' She had captured my attention now and I asked her what was that name again and she repeated it for me. I asked her to text me the name so I would not forget it and I continued stirring the pot. It had been an interesting but weird conversation at the same time. I waited two days for her to text me, but I received nothing and reluctantly I sent her a message: 'Hi Tameka, how you doing? Can you please remind me of that herb that your granddad takes for his diabetes that you told me about? Thanks, Lyndon.' She replied 18 minutes later.

Gradually my friends found out about my diabetes and they started to give me useful advice. At first, I was simply drinking water all day. This was a dramatic transition for me, not having tea or coffee with milk, sugar and honey and it was very tough, especially when I needed and wanted a refreshing drink, working all day in a hot kitchen.

I had an appointment to visit my friend, Prosper. Before my diabetes diagnosis, I used to have his walnut caramel cake, which was one of my favourites. On this visit, he said to me, 'Lyndon, do you want any cake? Please take one.' I thought, 'How can I say no to Lemon Tart - another of my favourites.'

Health Benefits of Spirulina

Nutrients*
Protein 12%
Calories 1%
Carbohydrate 1%
Fat 1%

Vitamins*
Riboflavin 20%
Thiamin 15%
Niacin 6%
Pantothenic Acid 3%

Minerals*
Copper 30%
Iron 15%
Manganese 9%
Magnesium 5%

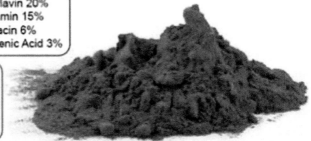

Helps to reduce ischemia and cholesterol levels

Gives relief from bronchial asthma

Beneficial for growth of probiotic bacteria, such as lactobacillus

Reduces kidney toxicity caused by chemotherapy

Effective in preventing growth of cancer

Aids in improving red blood cell count and boosts immune system

Provides protection against mercury poisoning

Helps to protect liver cells from toxin damage

Rich in immunomodulatory, antimicrobial and anti-inflammatory properties

Caution: Avoid giving spirulina to children without medical advice. Always buy it from a licensed and reputed manufacturer

*% Daily Value per 100g. For e.g. 100g of spirulina provides 30% of daily requirement of copper.

home remedies, with further information available from:

www.organicfacts.net

Spirulina is a natural 'algae' (cyanobacteria) powder that is incredibly high in protein and nutrients. When harvested correctly from non-contaminated ponds and bodies of water, it is one of the most potent nutrient sources available. It is largely made up of protein and essential amino acids and it is typically recommended for vegetarians because of its high natural iron content. It is often touted for its high vitamin B-12 content, though there is a lot of debate about if this particular form is a complete and absorbable form of B-12. It is not always recommended in place of animal products.

From a young age, the first time I tasted the Lemon Tart, I was hooked. There was something about that citrus smell and when it touched my tongue, it sent a tingle through my body, giving me an 'in the sky' feeling! However, that day with Prosper, we were in a general conversation but I remember my lips trembling when I said: 'I can't.' He replied, 'What do you mean, Lyndon? Why can't you?' I looked at him and said, 'I have type 2 diabetes'.

Instantly, the atmosphere changed. I said, jokingly, that I was not dying, but a lump came into my throat and I had to tell myself, 'Lyndon, take control.' Then he told me he was due to go for a blood test but was afraid of what his doctor might tell him. But he encouraged me by saying at least I got it checked out. I told him I had a scan on my stomach and told him I had a fatty liver.

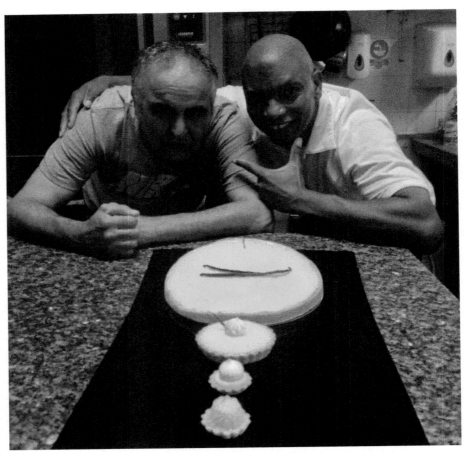

Lyndon with Prosper and his favourite Lemon Tarts

For the first time ever, I only took one cake home that day – for my wife, because I knew her weakness was the delicious Lemon Tart that I could not eat any more. Later that same day, at home, I asked my mother-in-law, 'Babcia, when you next go shopping, can you get me this spirulina please?' She took the note from me with the spelling of spirulina written on it, and within one minute she returned with a bottle of it. She had it in the kitchen cupboard and I had never recognised it nor seen it before.

My mother-in-law had a trace of breast cancer and she had researched natural food products. It was amazing because she also brought out chlorella powder for me. She had changed her diet and we simply let her get on with her healthy eating program and did not become involved. When I did more research for myself, I realised she had many of the food products already in the house that people were recommending to me and she saved me a lot of money.

However, taking spirulina is an acquired taste and one I found hard to adjust to at first when I tried it in water. The taste was disgusting and the smell off-putting as well. But my mother in-law was juicing carrots and she gave me some to add to hide the flavour! I like carrot juice and its natural sweetness so I put a teaspoon full of spirulina into it and drank it down; it was not nice! I started to add spirulina it to my porridge, which was surprisingly not too bad, and also sprinkling it onto other foods. Slowly and gradually, I accepted the taste and smell, because in my mind the benefits outweighed the dislikes.

A few days later, Tameka gave me more advice from her granddad. 'Lyndon, you should try drinking okra water, which is good for your liver.' I read up about this and it was the first thing I started to add to my daily water.

My cousin Dorothy introduced me to the benefits of cloves and I had not realised that we have been using cloves for years for its flavour rather than its medicinal benefits. I added it to my list of good foods and I added cloves to my Healthy Diabetic Cocktail – my daily drink.

When I received a text appointment reminder for the Chronic Disease Clinic, it upset me because it was the same address as my doctor's surgery and I thought they said I was simply seeing a dietician. I thought to myself, 'What have I got? Did they lie to me?' My appointment with the dietician was for 28 October. This was officially when I was informed that I had type 2 diabetes and that my HbA1c level was 92mmol/mol. As I waited at the surgery, I was anxious. But, when I was called in, I was greeted with a warm smile by the dietician.

Once in the room, she looked at the computer and said to me, 'Your HbA1c level is 92mmol/mol.' It didn't mean anything to me because I had never heard of this terminology before.

She went on to explain it was very high and the expression on her face made me more nervous and I remember feeling sick and uncomfortable. My heart started pumping fast and I felt myself starting to tremble while she continued looking at the computer screen. She told me directly, 'You will have to go on a drug called Metformin to help control your serious condition,' and she reached towards a huge pile of boxes on her desk.

It didn't mean much to me at that second, but as my lips trembled I remembered Ken's advice not to take any medication due to its potentially awful side effects. He had said to me, 'Make diet changes, take exercise and make sure you have an increased intake of flavonoid food instead of taking the medication you will be prescribed. When you take the tablets, you will never know if you are reducing your blood glucose levels because of the Metformin or because of the diet and exercise.'

I remember hearing myself say to the dietician, 'I want to try without Metformin.' She stopped talking for the first time in my appointment and actually looked at me. I think she agreed somewhat reluctantly. 'Alright,' she said, 'I will book you another blood test for Friday 13 November 2015, in 16 days' time.'

She said, 'We can test you in three months' time to see how you are getting on.' But I said, 'Let's keep it to the 16 days,' and we agreed. So she booked me in for the blood test and to see her 27 days later on Tuesday 24 November 2015, for a check-up.

She said I had to exercise and change my diet and recommended the four week NHS Diabetes Course entitled Starting Life With Diabetes and I agreed to attend. When we were finishing up, she seemed in a hurry for me to leave and quickly asked me how much I know about diabetes. She wrote down two websites for me to go to for more information. I left with a personal determination and a focused mindset to reduce my levels and get myself, my health and my body back into shape.

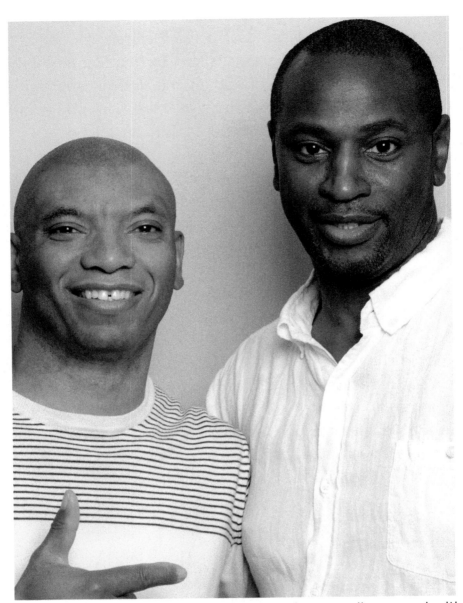

Lyndon with this cousin Ken Williams, who was diagnosed with type 1 diabetes in October 2013. Ken took medication for 19 months, before he reversed his condition and was able to stop taking the medication, from which he suffered bad side effects. Lyndon says, 'He is the reason I have reversed my diabetes in 105 days, without medication. Thank you, Ken, for your advice and recommendations, as well as your support and faith in me.'

Chapter 5

Crossing the Threshold and Committing to Change: going cold turkey

I thought to myself, 'I don't want these symptoms, the fear and the possibility of losing my ability to live life the way I do now, nor my livelihood nor my health,' and I simply decided to change my habits. I had my cousin Ken's experiences in my head and I simply went from eating and drinking massive amounts of sugar to having none. It was a black or white decision, a paradigm shift in my life, but I knew it was right for me, right now, before it was too late. I reset my mind and got on with it.

As I left the Chronic Disease Clinic that day, I was thinking of all the food I had to stop consuming, all those I loved best. I was off work for a couple of days and I stayed at home and wallowed in my misery, not really telling anyone except my wife. I was hiding, but actually I was also crossing a threshold in my life too. I was giving myself mental and physical space for my decision and its implications to sink in. I was committing to change in my way and my wife understood. I called Ken and told him what happened and my levels. He told me to start exercising, as well as changing my diet and he mentioned flavonoid food again.

The Importance of the Pancreas

Enzymes, or digestive juices, produced by the pancreas are secreted into the small intestine to further breakdown food after it has left the stomach. The gland also produces the hormone insulin and secretes it into the bloodstream to regulate the body's glucose or sugar level.

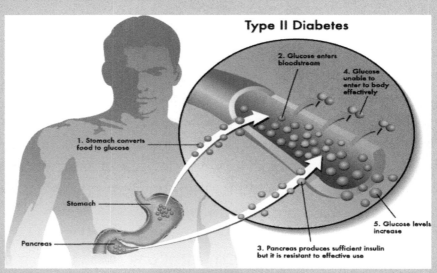

Type II Diabetes

1. Stomach converts food to glucose

2. Glucose enters bloodstream

4. Glucose unable to enter to body effectively

Stomach

Pancreas

5. Glucose levels increase

3. Pancreas produces sufficient insulin but it is resistant to effective use

The pancreas plays a crucial role in digestion. When food empties from your stomach into the small intestine, it mixes with digestive enzymes from the pancreas that neutralise stomach acid, preventing damage to the intestine. These enzymes also breakdown your food so your body can absorb it. The pancreas produces insulin, which reduces blood sugar levels and allows your body to store food energy for future use. Eating the right foods can heal and nourish your pancreas. It may also help you avoid pancreatitis, a painful inflammation of the pancreas.

I asked what these are with my focused interest now and he said they are food to help your condition, food that will help your pancreas and liver to recover, food such as dark chocolate and pears, which sounded alright to me! However, I wanted to know more about this diabetes and how to cure it. I was not thinking of reversing it, I wanted to cure it, and when I found out it was to do with the pancreas, I read up all I could find about the pancreas.

When I researched online, I discovered plenty of information and I realised why Ken had recommended I focus on eating flavonoid food and what brilliant advice he had given me. I started digging and digging for all the information I could find to reduce my sugar level. I trawled through diabetes websites, other people's stories, leaflets, brochures and books. I was like a learning sponge.

This gave me inspiration and fuelled my commitment to change and, of course, this research was invaluable for me! I want to share this invaluable information with you, and there is a chapter with more information coming in Chapter 6: Flavonoid Food and their Amazing Benefits: my secret weapon. This demonstrates the huge choice of food that becomes available to you when you start to look for alternatives and understand the benefits they each have for a healthier body.

After my big decision and my new focused mindset to achieve my goal of having a health body again, I started eating the following food, with reduced portions, on a regular basis.

Lyndon's Diet

Food

Poached eggs

Smoked turkey

Spirulina

Okra

Dark chocolate

Chlorella

Psyllium husk

Dragon fruit

Blueberries

Turmeric

Fenugreek

Fresh ginger

Red onions

Cloves

Fresh parsley

Grapefruit

Acai – super fruit juice

Fresh thyme

Kiwi

Cantaloupe melon

Sweet potato

Sunflower oil

Olive oil - extra virgin

Coconut oil – raw, organic, extra virgin

Wholemeal pasta

Brown rice

Brown basmati rice

Kale

Spinach

Broccoli

Cauliflower

Monkey nuts

Cod

Salmon

Smoked salmon

Grilled chicken

Red and yellow pepper

Baby gem lettuce

Drinks

Water

Lemon water

Cayenne pepper water

Ginger and lemon tea

Peppermint tea

Olive leaves tea

Cloves

Okra

Carrot juice

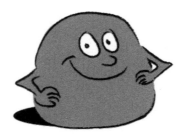

Billy the Blood Cell

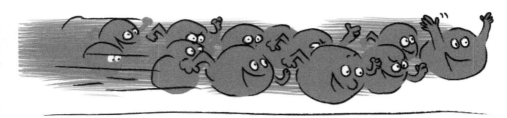

No glucose

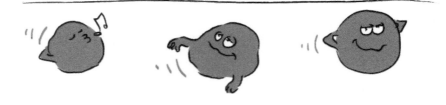

With glucose

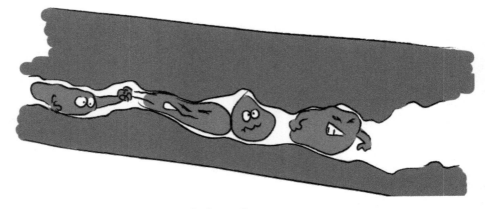

With plaque

What is the role of beta cells?

The pancreas contains beta cells, which release both insulin and glucagon. They are unique cells in the pancreas that produce, store and release the hormone insulin. Located in the area of the pancreas known as the islets of Langerhans (the organ's endocrine structures), they are one of at least five different types of islet cells that produce and secrete hormones directly into the bloodstream.

The main function of a beta cell is to produce and secrete insulin - the hormone responsible for regulating levels of glucose in the blood.

When blood glucose levels start to rise (e.g. during digestion), beta cells quickly respond by secreting some of their stored insulin while at the same time increasing production of the hormone.

This quick response to a spike in blood glucose usually takes about ten minutes.

In people with diabetes, however, these cells are either attacked or destroyed by the immune system (type 1 diabetes), or are unable to produce a sufficient amount of insulin needed for blood sugar control (type 2 diabetes).

Snacking Foods Before and After Diagnosis

Before Diagnosis	After Diagnosis
Crisps: Cheese and Onion, Prawn Cocktail, Salt and Vinegar, Smoked Chicken and Ready Salted	Fresh blueberries
Salted Peanuts	Monkey nuts
Chocolate bars: Kit Kats, Bounty,Wagon Wheel, Twix, Snickers	Smoked salmon with red onion and lemon juice on crackers
Biscuits: Chocolate Digestives, Custard Creams, Ritz Biscuits and Chocolate Chip Cookies	Avocado with red onion and lemon juice on crackers

Tuna fish with sweetcorn and lemon juice on crackers |
| Fizzy drinks and prune juice | Pears |
| | Dark chocolate |

The following facts can be researched online. They come from websites of many academic studies from around the world, which have discovered the benefits the following foods can have for people suffering from type 2 diabetes.

Cayenne Pepper

Cayenne pepper and other chilli powders have been a traditional treatment for diabetes for many years.

Ginger

Ginger can increase uptake of glucose into muscle cells without using insulin.

Cinnamon

Cinnamon may reduce risk factors associated with diabetes and cardiovascular disease. The scientific evidence available, and many health experts, claim that cinnamon contains properties beneficial for blood sugar regulation.

Lemon Water

The sour taste of lemon is due to the presence of 5% to 6% of citric acid in lemon juice. This distinctive taste of lemon juice also makes it one of the important ingredients either when it is used in drinks or food such as cocktails, lemonade and soft drinks.

Lemon juice can also be used as a preservative for certain foods, which oxidise and turn brown after they are sliced, such as apples, bananas and avocados.

Cloves

Cloves come from a flower bud of a tropical evergreen tree. Research promotes the use of cloves for patients with diabetes for the glucose-lowering impacts experienced when consuming cloves on a daily basis.

Snacking

Before being diagnosed, I was snacking on foods all the way through the day. However, since my diagnosis, I have discovered even more foods that I can snack on and enjoy, which are good for me and are nourishing my liver and my pancreas at the same time. More flavoursome options opened up for me when I did my research and I learnt more about it.

I also ate a lot of blueberries, which I learnt have terrific benefits as a food for diabetics. Not only are blueberries a really good fruit for diabetics, the good news for Black men is that prostate cancer can be warded off by a healthy dose of blueberries in your diet. The vitamin C, vitamin A and phytonutrients in blueberries have powerful antioxidants that protect your cells from tumour growth and inflammation. The foliate in blueberries also serves as synthesis and repair agents, stopping the formation of cancer cells from growing and spreading. Throat, lung, mouth, pharynx, endometrial, pancreatic and colon cancer all benefit from the bluest eye of fruits.

If you're having trouble getting back and forth to the toilet with a regular stool, blueberries are the secret to get your bowels moving.

That powerful thing called fibre is responsible for preventing constipation and keeping your digestive tract in tip-top shape.

If you are on a diet and are always feeling hungry at the end of a meal, try eating blueberries. The fibre inside the blueberries increases satiety and reduces your appetite.

The studies also show that blueberries contain phytonutrient antioxidants that protect your eyes from oxidative stress. This fruit also protects your retina from sunlight damage.

Blueberries are perfect snacks for the morning, lunch and dinner. Whether you're eating them whole, in a fresh juice or as an additive to your salad, blueberries are a great way to improve your overall health.

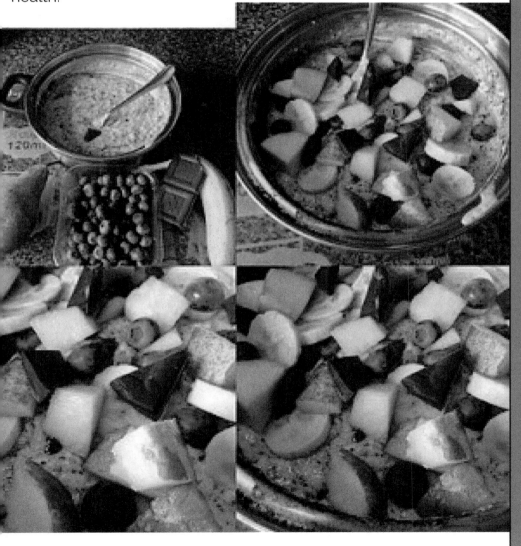

A Fasting Chef!

Many years ago, some friends and I challenged each other to have a 24-hour no-food fast after going through a session of talking about health and well-being. None of us had ever done this before and it was a challenge we took seriously. I must admit, that for me it was a long and tough 24 hours. I remember being really hungry and having feelings and bodily reactions I had never felt before. I survived the hunger pains and the wanting to eat all the way through the day, but the best aspect that I learnt about myself was that if I did not concentrate on it, I did not feel the hunger quite so badly!

As the hours counted down and at the glorious moment of the 24-hour mark, I thought I would be ravenously hungry and all day I had been thinking about the food I will break my fast with. But when the time came to eat, I felt fine and not as desperate to eat as I thought I would be! It was a bit of an anti-climax, especially because if I was hungry I would have eaten something substantial.

My experiences as a chef working in different establishments are that each kitchen has its own routines. In some places, a chef has a lunch break, and in some other places lunch is provided for all staff.

Work lunch options I have experienced include:

- eating at normal lunch times as customers or other work colleagues between 12pm and 1pm;
- after the lunch service in a restaurant or in a banqueting kitchen at about 2pm;
- no lunch provided by the chef of the establishment and chefs bring in their own lunch;
- not being able to snack as you work throughout the morning; and
- not offering staff any food by the chef of an establishment.

These are aspects that chefs have to cope with, sometimes with no food throughout the day, although being surrounded by food all day.

In hindsight, this has put me in the position of being able to be mentally and physically prepared to fast for up to six hours, 12 hour and 24 hours, having only water. On other occasions and in some kitchens, it is normal to snack on fruits, biscuits, cakes, bread, meat and cake trimmings that are in the kitchen.

During the period of reversing my diabetes, I was so conscious of every piece of food I was putting into my mouth, that when I was around food I knew I was not supposed to eat, I drank only water. I had days when I didn't want to eat anything to keep the sugar levels down.

These were mentally tough days, but I had set my goals to reduce the levels. I knew this was a temporary situation so this was a highly motivating factor for me to fast.

The most frequent times I did a 24-hour fast, only drinking water, was when I knew I had a blood test the next day. Now I can pick and choose when to fast and it has become part of my nutrition strategy. For example, I use fasting as a healing and cleansing program when I allow myself to eat too much on special occasions, I fast the next day to balance out my weekly intake.

The importance of waist measurement

Waist measurement is especially important if you are a diabetic. When we carry excess weight around our middle, 'apple shaped', we are more at risk of high blood pressure and heart disease than those people who carry excess weight around their bottom and thighs, 'pear shaped'.

With diabetes, excess weight around the middle increases insulin resistance. This means our bodies cannot use its own insulin properly and extra glucose stays in our blood rather than being used by our body. The great news is that even a small reduction in waist measurement can make a big difference to improving health!

My Tips to Help You

Find your waist measurement and check the table below to see if you are at risk. These figures are provided by the UK's National Health Service and measurements can very slightly depending on your ethnicity.

Measuring your waist is easy. Find the bottom of your ribs and the top of your pelvis bone and measure around your middle at the point halfway between these two. For most people, it is at the level of your tummy button or slightly above. It is important you do not hold your tummy in or wear any belts or tight waistbands while taking your waist measurement. Lifestyle changes, including changing your diet and taking up a regular exercise regime, can help reduce those inches around your middle and reduce your risk. It makes sense. Just do it!

Ideal Waist Measurement

	Healthy	At Risk	Great Risk
Women	23.5 inches 60 – 80 cm	31.5 – 34.5 inches 80 – 88 cm	+ 34.5 inches + 88 cm
Men	27.5 – 37 inches 69 – 94 cm	37 – 40 inches 94 – 102 cm	+ 40 inches + 102 cm

NHS Recommendations provided by the Buckinghamshire Healthcare Trust, January 2016

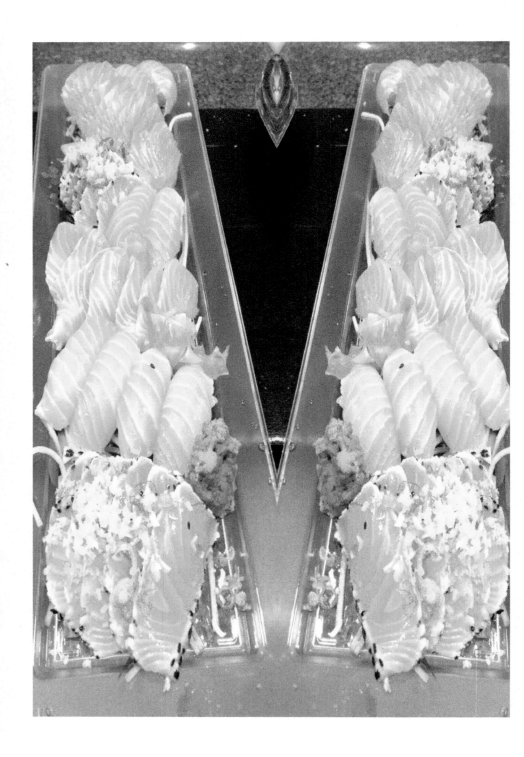

Chapter 6:
Flavonoid Food and their Amazing Benefits: my secret weapon!

From all the research I completed and the advice I was given by my family and friends, I learnt that there are more than 6,000 food and drinks identified as flavonoid food. This chapter shares with you the information about flavonoid food which I discovered during my recovery. Knowing about these food groups will help you improve and widen the range of your diet, as I did. You can do further research about these food and their benefits.

Flavonoid food are a diverse group of phytonutrients produced by plants and they are our greatest source of healthy nutrients. Among all the plant food groups, it has always been fruits and vegetables that have been best studied and most analysed for their flavonoid content. There is also flavonoid data on nuts and seeds, grains, beans and vegetables and other foods and drinks, including green and black tea. From my online research about flavonoid food, I found the most useful information from the U.S. Department of Agriculture's (USDA) Flavonoid Database. Here they actually breakdown the flavonoid analyses into five of the basic flavonoid chemical subgroups and analyse the best food choices in each of these subgroups. This is a useful approach to understanding the flavonoid content of food, because it emphasises the need to eat a wide variety of flavonoids that includes all of the different types.

Best Sources of Flavonoids

The information below will help you learn about the top World Health Food in each of the five flavonoid subcategories. When I discovered this information, I realised why Ken had recommended I focus on eating flavonoid food and what brilliant advice he had given me.

Provided by Whole Foods Market, America's Healthiest Grocery Store, for further details visit: ww.wholefoodsmarket.com/

Flavonols	Flavan-3-ols*	Flavones	Flavonones	Anthocyanidins
Onions	Apples	Parsley	Oranges	Blueberries
Apples	Bananas	Bell peppers	Grapefruit	Bananas
Romaine lettuce	Blueberries	Celery	Lemons	Strawberries
Tomatoes	Peaches	Apples	Tomatoes	Cherries
Garbanzo beans	Pears	Oranges		Pears
Almonds	Strawberries	Watermelon		Cabbage
Turnip greens		Chilli peppers		Cranberries
Sweet potatoes		Cantaloupe melon		Plums
Quinoa		Lettuce		Raspberries
				Garbanzo beans

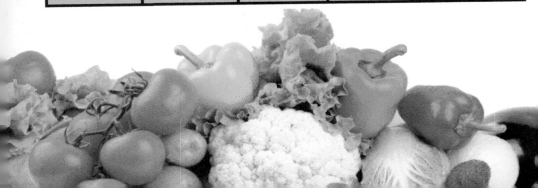

Food source	Flavones	Flavonols	Flavanones
Red onion	0	4 – 100	0
Parsley, fresh	24 - 634	8 - 10	0
Thyme, fresh	56	0	0
Lemon juice, fresh	0	0 – 2	2 – 175

As well as all the naturally good, healthy food and drink I have already mentioned, which helped me to cure my type 2 diabetes, on the following pages are the flavonoid food options, which you can now select from and enjoy.

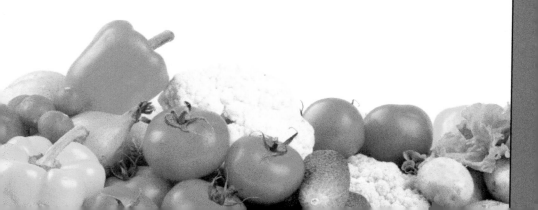

Blueberries and Cherries

Blueberries and cherries are good sources of antioxidants, which help prevent cell damage.

Cruciferous vegetables - general

Broccoli and other cruciferous vegetables, including brussel sprouts, cabbage, cauliflower, kohlrabi, turnips and red cabbage. They contain powerful chemicals, which may help prevent cancer.

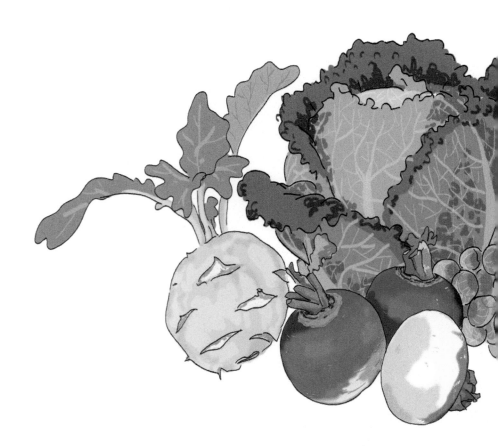

Garlic

Garlic and onions are a good source of beneficial nutrients for a healthy pancreas.

Red Grapes

Red grapes are a powerful antioxidant. Avoid red wine if you have pancreatitis and eat a handful of red grapes instead.

Red Reishi Mushrooms

Red reishi mushrooms can help reduce inflammation and are used in Chinese medicine to restore balance to the body.

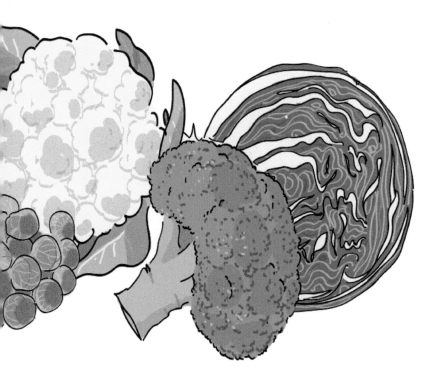

Spinach

Spinach is a great source of iron and vitamin B, which your pancreas needs. Try a spinach salad, or spinach stir-fried with garlic. Other leafy greens, including kale, mustard and Swiss chard are also beneficial for your pancreas.

Sweet Potatoes

Sweet potatoes, as well as other Beta-carotene orange and yellow vegetables, including, carrots, corn and squash, contain nutrients, which are beneficial for the pancreas and can help prevent cancer.

Tofu

Tofu is an excellent source of low-fat protein. You need protein in your diet for healing, but too much fat will exacerbate any pancreas problems.

Tomato Vegetable Soup

Tomatoes are a great source of vitamin C and antioxidants. Vegetables also contain antioxidants and beneficial nutrients and soup provides additional fluid.

Yogurt with Active Cultures

Yogurt with active cultures is a great source of probiotics, beneficial bacteria, which help keep the immune and digestive system functioning at their best. Choose yogurt with no sugar.

Cayenne Pepper

Many societies, especially those of the Americas and China, have a history of using cayenne pepper therapeutically. A powerful compound with many uses, cayenne pepper is gaining popularity as a cleansing and detoxifying food, which stimulates the circulation and neutralises acidity. It is also used these days in detoxification because it increases the body's ability to sweat. Cayenne tea is an excellent morning beverage when you want to detox and lose weight.

Cayenne is known as a great metabolic booster, aiding the body to burn excess amounts of fats. It is also a useful ingredient for diabetics because it helps to keep blood pressure levels normalised and can help balance the body of bad cholesterol and triglycerides.

Historically, cayenne pepper has been used to heal many ailments including heartburn, delirium, tremors, gout, paralysis, fever, dyspepsia, flatulence, sore throat, atonic dyspepsia, haemorrhoids, menorrhagia in women, nausea, tonsillitis, scarlet fever and diphtheria. It is known to have many health benefits and I recommend you research these further and use it for yourself.

Spirulina

Spirulina offers many health benefits for diabetics including: lowering cholesterol levels; enhancing immunity; increasing red blood cell count; providing anti-cancerous properties and anti-inflammatory properties; protecting the liver; reducing the toxicity in the kidneys; controlling bronchial asthma; and enhancing the supply of antioxidants.

Spirulina is a blue-green algae named after its perfect spiral shape and it belongs to a cyanobacteria species. It is scientifically known as *Arthrospira platensis*. It is generally found in alkaline lakes in Mexico and Africa and is rich in nutrients, including proteins, carbohydrates, vitamins, minerals and trace elements.

This amazing food first came to light in the 1940s in French Equatorial Africa, when French troops stumbled on a food the locals were growing. It was growing on the surface of lakes and being collected, sun-dried and sold in the local markets. Biologists concluded that it was an algae being grown and eaten. Spirulina is also the food choice of local birds, such as flamingoes.

Historical writings show it was consumed as food during the time of the Spanish conquest during the 15th century. Columbus' personal literature revealed something about an ooze-like substance being collected from lakes, sun-dried and baked like bread.

Spirulina is also well-known as one of the highest sources of protein. It is also a good source of vital micronutrients, is easily digested and is beneficial for probiotic bacteria, such as lactobacillus, which live inside our digestive system.

Spirulina is the richest plant source for Beta-carotene and phycocyanin, which are biochemicals with anti-cancerous properties. It is known to help in significantly controlling liver cancer.

However, nutrient supplements, including Spirulina, can interact with medications and should only be taken after discussion with your doctor. Spirulina can sometimes be contaminated with heavy metals that can be toxic. Therefore, buying it from a licensed and reputed manufacturer is advised. Always avoid giving Spirulina to children without medical advice.

Okra

Okra is fast gaining a reputation as a so-called superfood for people with or at risk of diabetes or cancer. It is more commonly referred to as ladyfingers, or by its biological names *Abelmoschus esculentus and Hibiscus esculentus*. Okra is known to have a positive effect on blood sugar control, among many other health benefits. It is a tall-growing, green vegetable that traces its origin from ancient Ethiopia (Abyssinia) through to Eastern Mediterranean, India, the Americas and the Caribbean. Parts of the plant (immature okra pods) are widely used as vegetables in tropical countries and are typically used for making soups, stews or as a fried and boiled vegetable.

Psyllium Husks

The soluble fibre found in psyllium husks can help to lower cholesterol. Psyllium can also help to relieve constipation and diarrhoea and is used to treat irritable bowel syndrome, haemorrhoids and other intestinal problems. Psyllium has also been used to help regulate blood sugar levels in diabetics.

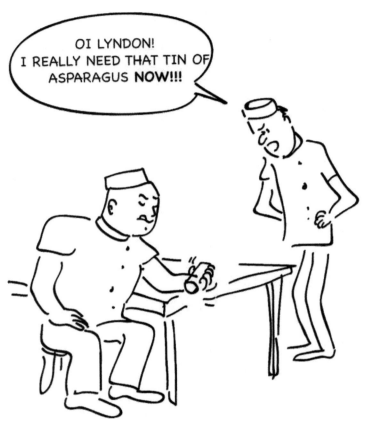

Lyndon doing his morning exercises

CHAPTER 7

Enjoying Exercise: starting in the gym!

Marlon Mellish of Will2Win, who represented England as a lightweight boxer and participated in more than 45 amateur fights, told me that the benefits of exercise for diabetes sufferers include:

- reduces insulin sensitivity;
- lowers blood pressure;
- reduces body fat; and
- lowers risk of heart disease.

Ivan, a chef I was working with, started riding his bike to work and eating more healthy food. After a period of time, I saw a difference in his body.

He was losing weight and I saw the positive change in him and I thought to myself, 'I need to get on my bike.' I had this vision of me moving all the stuff in the garden shed where my bike was covered in cobwebs behind the chairs and garden hose!

But I knew I had to take some sensible exercise and so I did take my bike out and went for a morning ride with my wife.

I hadn't ridden my bike out for months before that, but it was fun and I felt good afterwards! It played on my mind that I needed to be doing more exercise or something physical. I took out the leather skipping rope and hung it up on the wall to stretch it out over the living room door because the leather was normally tangled. But that was the end of that - my mother-in-law took it down again to tidy up the room and folded it away and put it back to its tangled self!

But I knew that not taking exercise was one of my biggest challenges and so I decided I needed to go to the gym and I booked an induction at my local gym in November 2015. My lack of exercise had always played on my mind. The determination was there, but the action was slow, overthinking what was the best exercise for me.

I enjoyed my induction and went straight into action and found my routine using the cross trainer, bike, rowing machine, back extensions, leg raises and other muscle building machines. Actually, I was reminiscing back to my days as a youth in the gym, but whatever it took to make me do it was good!

After I had signed up at the gym, my idea was only to lose weight. I established a good routine of dropping off my daughter at school, going to the gym up to three times per week and drinking a bottle of water afterwards back in the car. I also ate a punnet of blueberries and a banana, before going off to do my chores or go to work.

I wondered what else I could do and so I registered with the Wycombe 50 Plus Club. It is a funny story actually because when I went to see what classes they offered, they did not believe that

I was old enough to join them! As I was looking at the leaflets on the table, a man sitting there acknowledged me and asked how he could help me. I asked how to join up but he said, 'Why do you need to join? You don't look 50.' But I said, 'I am 50,' and he smiled and giggled. Another man came to the desk and they both exchanged greetings and giggled in my direction so I took out my driving license and showed them. They couldn't believe it, as I filled out the joining application form. The man said there is a waiting list before you can participate in any activities. Two weeks later, they called me and said I can come to the next session but by then I had lost interest because I was enjoying the gym, although I liked the idea of the group cycling!

My gym routine went on until the gym shut down a few months after I joined, but my mind was made up and fortunately there was a sister gym a few miles away, which was also available to us. It felt like a bit of a distance, but by this time I had caught the bug and had to go, so I did.

My friend Bogdan gave me some heartfelt advice to increase the benefits from my exercise routine, after I told him I was going to the gym. He told me to start with 25 minutes on the cross trainer machine. I found it hard to do 15 minutes and actually it started to hurt after only five minutes, but I respected Bogdan's advice and I progressed slowly.

I started adding five minutes on the cross trainer each time I went to the gym. It felt good and I enjoyed the exercise and the sense of achievement it gave me.

Ivan had introduced me to psyllium husk a long time ago and in November I bought some to try. However, as I sat drinking water in the car after my gym workout, I remember thinking how nice it would be to have a tall glass of lemonade, just like we used to in the early days of my career.

The Savoy Hotel.
London

No 4876   16th May   1986

This is to Certify that

LYNDON WISSART

has been employed by The Savoy Hotel, London,

in Restaurant Kitchen

as Apprentice Chef, 2nd Commis II.

from 28th August *19* 84 *to* 16th May   *19* 86

During his employment with The Savoy, Mr Wissart carried out his

duties to the best of his ability and proved to be a loyal,

reliable employee. He leaves of his own accord and can be

recommended.

Head of the Department.   *General Manager.*

Signature of the holder of this Certificate.

Flashback Two:

The Savoy Hotel and the influences of my early career

I went to school at Drayton Secondary School, London where I found out about the Youth Training Scheme. It was a vocational training system in the 1970s, which provided on-the-job training for school leavers, aged 16 and 17, across a wide range of hospitality sectors. I successfully got myself through several interviews and by the time I was signed up on the scheme, I discovered I had been selected out of about 2,000 candidates. I remember feeling good about myself then. The scheme allowed us to work in different hotel departments including: accounts, banqueting, room service, reception and the enquiries desk for the first 12 months. After that, we had to choose which department we wanted to work in, which meant there was a guaranteed job at the end of the scheme.

It sounded good to me as an ambitious teenager, and I started at the Mount Royal Hotel in Marble Arch, London. I enjoyed the training and I remember once we went for a team building trip to Wales, where we abseiled and tried crossbow distance shooting, which I won much to my surprise! We also had a go at canoeing and taking part in a map reading exercise to find hidden objects. It was a fun week with friends who were in the same place as me.

I had always wanted to be a chef and it was an easy choice for me to select the kitchen to work in; I went straight into the Grill Restaurant at the Mount Royal Hotel. I was excited to have a job to do and I was motivated to do it well.

My desire to become a chef had started at a young age, when my parents gave me my first house key with a threaded string with bits hanging off it. I remember it well because it meant I could let myself into the house when no one else was there. This gave me my first taste of responsibility, because if I was alone in the house when I got back from school, it meant I had to cook something to eat because I was hungry.

My mother always grew scallion in our garden; this is what she called them being from the West Indies, while in the UK we know them as spring onions. I would pick them, wash them, fry them and add baked beans, just like my mother did. In this way, I started experimenting with the different foods in the house and my passion for cooking grew naturally. When it came to choosing 5th form school subjects, which in those days were a choice of: Needlework; Metal Work; Woodwork; Biology; French; Social Studies; or Home Economics (cooking), my first choice was obviously Home Economics.

However, I was the first and only boy in a class of all girls, until a boy called David joined us later on. After a while, some of the girls in the class asked me for help or advice, so I guess I must have been doing something right even then!

My second job after the Mount Royal Hotel was at Hamleys Toy Shop on Regent Street, where I worked in the restaurant for two months before securing a great job at the Savoy Hotel on the

Strand. I started at the Savoy Hotel as an apprentice chef on the hot fish section. But actually I worked my way through all the different sections, including: cold fish; roast; larder; sauce; and vegetables, before I was promoted to commis chef, as it was called in those days in a proper kitchen. In fact, I was fortunate because I was fast tracked and this gave me a good start in my professional career as a high-quality chef. Although I was working as a commis chef, I was also given the role as a chef de partie, where you oversee a section of the kitchen. This included pastry, butchery, fish, sauces, vegetables and is why the job is sometimes called a station chef or line cook. In large kitchens, you usually have help from a demi-chef de partie, commis or trainee chef.

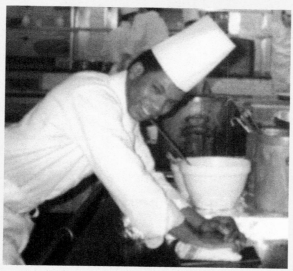

The Savoy Hotel has much memorable history for me and I remember my first day in the kitchen, when I walked in and there was a lot of noise. Everyone seemed to be shouting with food orders coming from all directions and being amplified through a loud speaker system, in words I had never heard before! 'Oui, chef'; 'on comune'; 'champignons'; 'envoyer appartement' etc. I did not understand a word because it was all in French, but straight into the fire I went boldly!

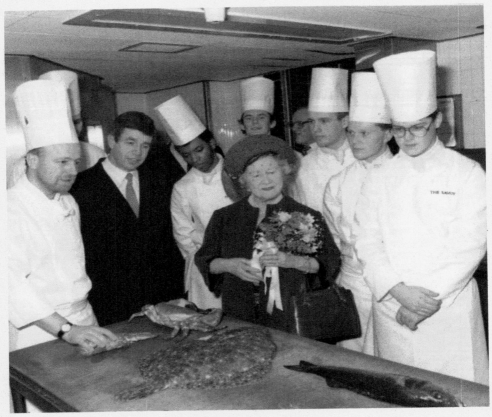

Courtesy The Savoy
**The Queen Mother admiring fish in the Savoy kitchen with
head chef Anton Edelmann, commis chef Lyndon Wissart and
other staff.**

The head chef Anton Edelmann introduced me to David Sharlan, who was to be my mentor on the hot fish section. I started as I mentioned as a trainee chef at the Savoy but I was very quickly doing the job as chef de partie at the same time. This was huge leap for a young man like me. I was only 20 years old. In layman's term, I was running a section: such as hot fish; cold fish; roast; and sauce; well before my time, and also attending chef de partie meetings as a commis.

I had huge opportunities for learning and I grabbed them all and developed my skills in the kitchen every week. I still have a lot of respect for Anton Edelmann, a man who believed in me and gave me the opportunity to grow as a chef. I acknowledge him and thank him for all he taught me and the many opportunities he gave him at such a young age. I was always eager to learn and he saw that and encouraged and challenged me, which I loved and responded well to.

The kitchen was extremely hot, like a furnace. Heat I have never felt before; the stoves were heated by coal so the heat from the stovetop in front of you was intense as you worked to cook the fish orders. After the service and the last orders were called, we had to clean the top of the stoves using a brick or something similar wrapped in sand paper and the only way to get it clean was to scrub the hot steel top until it was shiny.

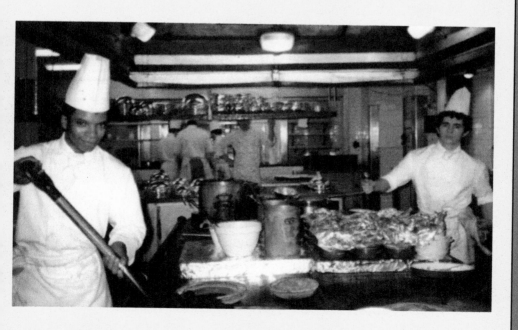

After the service was over, we all went in our chef whites to change and wash up but we always ended up covered in black marks from the coal and from being drenched with sweat. The first time I looked into the mirror, I saw black marks around my eyes and on my eyelids, in my nostrils, and in and behind my ears, and I remember having black fingernails between the nail and skin. I used to touch it and rub it between my fingers. It was a black sandy texture to my surprise, but it was the coal dust that came from the cooker's solid tops and it got all over us chefs!

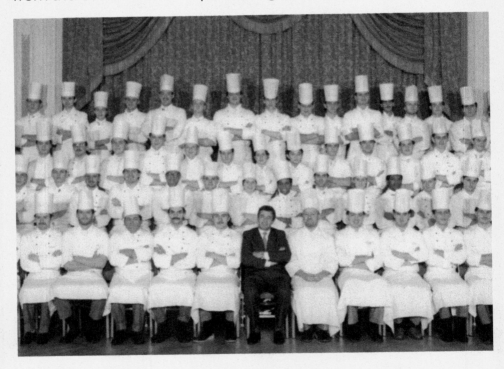

During and after the food service, I was always dying of thirst for a drink, and water or lemonade was available. I always chose the lemonade of course, because it was a luxury drink, and because as a child my family could not afford these luxuries. When the trolley of lemonade came around, my eyes opened up with joy and we were able to drink as much as we liked!

The chefs were given lemonade to drink because it was so hot in the kitchen and the management wanted to keep us happy and energised.

However, one day, I consumed so much lemonade, I can remember having stomach pains and I could hardly walk. I was leaning against the corridor wall. Mr Edelmann questioned me and then sent me home, saying I needed to see a doctor. After being examined and answering all his questions, I was diagnosed with gastroenteritis.

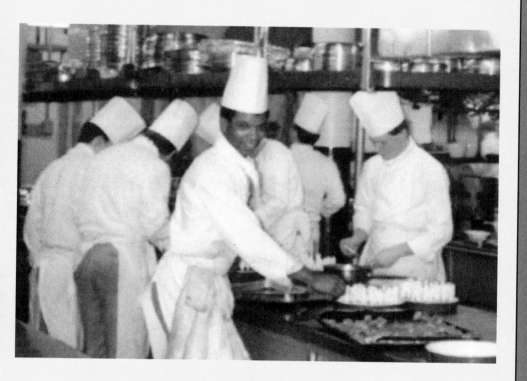

Flashback Three:

1990s - my relationship with sugar had even more serious consequences than I could have ever believed. In the 1990s, when I was in my thirties, a young man at the peak of my life, I was always tired and everywhere I went I was known to sleep very easily. I would rest my head whenever I could and doze off! It was very unusual for a young man normally so full of eager energy, but I could not control it. I became well known for this and people would say, 'I hope you are not going to sleep,' whenever I was visiting them!

However, it was just how I was, but I did not realise the masses amounts of sugar that I was consuming every day, not only from the food I ate, but also from the drinks I loved too! At this point, I was probably pre-diabetic without knowing about it.

Alcohol was always in the home and it was nice to have a sip now and again with my family. The reason for having so much alcohol was we had plenty of family and friends visiting and bringing a drink to celebrate the birth of my twin children.

As we are of West Indian descent, this was a regular occurrence and I was consuming alcohol combined with a high carbohydrate diet, which of course turns into sugar in the body. It must have been having a detrimental effect on my system, but I did not know about it then! I was a young father with three children under the age of five and I was a consistent drinker - we had much to celebrate!

At this time in my life, I was eating and drinking whatever I wanted without worrying about it nor really thinking about it. I was a chef and I knew about nutrition and food and so there was no reason to question my habits, or was there? Looking back, I can see the pattern of ill health had set in, but I did not realise it at the time.

I used to start my day with a cup of tea in the morning, with two teaspoons of sugar in it and I ate at least three slices of toast with butter and jam. Sometimes for breakfast at home, I cooked three fried eggs, bacon, baked beans and fried onions. Alternatively, it was three eggs, sausages, fried onions, fried tomatoes, baked beans, with two rashers of bacon, ham and two slices of bread.

I remember sometimes having a cup of tea during and after eating breakfast and feeling sick afterwards. It was an uncomfortable feeling. Even though at times I knew I was going to feel this way, I still had the tea because I enjoyed the taste so much.

In my car on the way to work, I always ate and drank: tea in the morning in a flask with three teaspoons of demerara sugar with honey, and three slices of toast with strawberry jam. I also ate Honey and Oat Crunchy and I had a box of 24 in my car boot, so I never ran out! I also sometimes ate biscuits or homemade cakes.

When I got to work, as I mentioned earlier, I had another breakfast, of golden syrup flavoured porridge, to which I added honey. I drank coffee made from a latte sachet, with lots of milk and I would add sugar and honey. I also sometimes ate digestive biscuits, one of my favourites, and I snacked on cake trimmings all the way through the day!

At lunchtime at work, I usually ate a curry meal of onion bhaji from the local shop or homemade food in the kitchen, something the chefs made for all the staff. With my lunch, I drank J20 apple and raspberry juice, Kia, mango juice, basil seed drink, aloe vera drink or super malt.

Fortunately, I was in the habit of taking supplements, which had a positive effect on me, because what I was taking were good for diabetics, not that I knew anything about diabetes at that time of my life!

The supplements I took included:

- Lutein and Zeaxanthin;
- Omega 3;
- Vitamin C;
- Bilberry;
- Beta-carotene;
- Ginkgo and Ginseng;
- Saw Palmetto; and
- Multivitamins.

I consumed a fizzy drink, or chocolate bar, or packet of crisps in the car. At home I ate whatever was around, from a snack, takeaway, healthy meal or a quick fry-up. Sometimes I ate for the sake of eating, although I was not really hungry.

Chapter 8 -

Suffering a Christmas Setback: my low point and 'Excusitis!'

It was December 2015, with Christmas coming and I was working long hours, although it was beginning to be time for family and friends, but I had to stay focused on my work.

For my Christmas present, my wife bought me an Accu-Chek, a mobile glucose testing monitor. I thought it was a great gift and I sent my cousin Ken a photo boastfully saying look what I had got given for Christmas. His reply was, 'You know they are free on the NHS (smiley face with sweat),' I replied, 'Try telling my dietician! (emoji face).'

Christmas in my family is always an exciting time, with fun games and, of course, good food and plenty to drink. I had made a banana cake and carrot cake for a friend and I doubled the recipe and made extra for us. However, during this happy, holiday period, I suffered a major setback because I relaxed and overindulged. I ate and drank too many sweet foods and drinks. I realised what was happening and started to weigh myself two or three times a day. Our weighing scales were easily available in the bathroom and I discovered I had put on a kilo of weight and my glucose level rose to 11.9!

I knew I had to recharge my motivation and refocus my mindset and to get back on track after the holidays. I was going to have to work hard to maintain the effect of the progress I had made previously. Fortunately, I thought back to a book that influenced me when I was young. It gave me that flash of focus I needed right at that moment in my life, to reignite my thinking on my goal to get rid of these symptoms, keep my levels low and be truly healthy.

I found this book highly motivational, *The Magic of Thinking Big* by David Schwartz, especially, his 'Excusitis' chapter, which really helped me on my journey.

PART THREE:
MODERATION

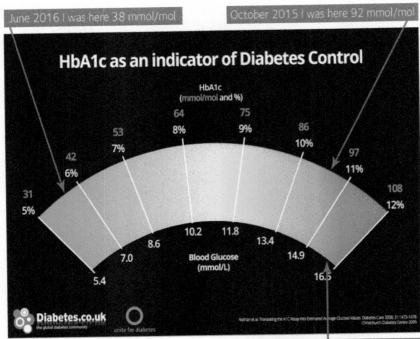

What is HbA1c?

The term *HbA1c* refers to glycated haemoglobin. It develops when haemoglobin, a protein within red blood cells that carries oxygen throughout your body, joins with glucose in the blood, becoming 'glycated'. By measuring glycated haemoglobin (HbA1c), clinicians are able to get an overall picture of what our average blood sugar levels have been over a period of weeks/months.

Date	Blood Glucose Level	Weight lose	HbA1C Results	Impact
October 2015	15.9	85/86 kilos, 13.5 stone	92 mmol/mol	Serious type 2 diabetes
November 2015		83 Kilos, 13 stone	77 mmol/mol	Bad type 2 diabetes
December 2015 9th December, 26th December	5.9, 11.9	81 Kilos, 12.5 stone	60 mmol/mol	Average type 2 diabetes
1st February 2016		81 Kilos, 12.5 Stone	41 mmol/mol	Normal type 2 diabetes
29 Febuary 2016		77.5 Kilos, 12 stone	39 mmol/mol	Cured controlled reversed
8 June 2016		75.8 kilos, 11 stone	38 mmol/mol	Reversed and feeling amazing!
19 October 2016		76 kilos, 11.8 stone	36 mmol/mol	Reversed and still feeling amazing!

 @lwissart   lwissart   lwissart   lwissart

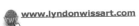 www.lyndonwissart.com

Chapter 9:

Rededication to Change; and diabetes courses

I remember after Christmas, in January 2016, I went shopping - not the usual type - because I had a list of flavonoid food to purchase. This was my first and focused thought. I needed to be eating the right foods to heal and nourish my pancreas and also to reduce my blood sugar levels.

I went to food supplement shops to find special dietary foods for diabetics. I specifically wanted a healthy replacement for honey because honey was one of my favourite healthy sweeteners. I found one but when I read the label, I had my doubts. So I did not use it; instead I took it with me to the first diabetic course to check with the dietician.

A new gym had opened in Wycombe, so I went to take a look and see what I thought. The new gym gave me and my wife a free induction. It was really exciting with a special feeling in the air as we walked the newly built premises. There was clean air and a spotless floor, the size of the leisure centre that we had been going to before. We were met by the friendly gym staff who led us to the immaculate gym where we had to put on blue shoe covers because it was all sparkling new. We went into the gym, where the size was overwhelming.

The amount of new and different types of machines was amazing and we had the opportunity to try them out, which was fun, especially together. I was excited and looking forward to getting back into my gym routine.

The next day, I was back at the new gym and focused on getting back into my routine as fast as possible. I knew I had the time to do this and I knew how important it was for my health and to achieve my goal. I stayed for one hour, really enjoying using all the new machines and being in such a pristine environment. It felt good to be back and doing something practical to help my health.

There were new classes to join and new equipment to use and of course, a new 50 Plus Club. After looking at the classes, I thought I would try the cycling class, since it was a new event. On my way to the registration table, a short wrinkly 50 plus lady came up to me and stopped me in my stride and asked if she can help me. I replied, 'I am just looking at what classes are scheduled and what I have to do to join.' She said, 'This is a 50 Plus Club,' and I said, ;I know,' – 'Here we go again,' I thought to myself! She said, 'You're not 50,' and I just looked at her. 'How old do you think I am?' She said, 'About 35,' Another lady standing next to her said, 'You have no wrinkles.' So with my cheeky sense of humour, I asked them, 'Do you have to have wrinkles to be 50 years old?' But then I was more polite and I offered to show them my ID and I told them that I had registered in 2015 but did not attend any classes. The first lady told me that my name will have been taken off the list and there is a waiting list so it may take time for you to be able join. I did put my name down to join, but this second encounter about my age made me feel good. Maybe my change of diet and exercise had made me look even younger than last time I had tried to join the 50 Plus Club!

I told my cousin Ken excitedly about my progress, but asked him why I didn't sweat much in the gym. He gave me this glaring look, implying there must be something wrong with me. He asked me what my heart rate was on the machines I was using. But I didn't know because I had never looked or thought about it. He told me to raise my heart rate to about 140 and I would start sweating. The next time I went on the cross trainer, I keyed in for the heart rate program, but no heart rate was showing. Was I dead? No, very much alive! I cancelled the program and started again. This time, I followed the instructions more carefully, putting my hands on the shiny metal handles, and after a few seconds, up came my low heart rate.

'Alright,' I said to myself, 'Lyndon, let's step this up., I put up the resistance and started pushing away. It was tough but I had my goal set and I had something to aim for, my motivation factor. I slowly felt the sweat building up and getting ready to roll down the side of my face and when it did, the feeling of achievement came rushing through my body. I set my next goal to maintain it and I got it up to the 140 heart rate target. I kept the pressure on, maintaining and going above 140, 143, 145. It got to an amazing 150. It felt real and rewarding. 'Is this me?' I said to myself. I got to the stage where I could not maintain it anymore, I felt the wind knocked out of my lungs and I watched the heart rate steadily drop down back to a steady, slower pace, but at least I had achieved my heart rate goal of 140. Since that experience, I use this as my benchmark target, but it was hard to maintain and became my progressing challenge.

However, I felt really good being back at the gym and I had found my routine and kept on track as the new year - 2016 - progressed! After trying all the new machines, I found a routine I was comfortable with, including using the cross trainer, bike, rowing machine, the lateral machine and vibrating machine. However, I decided to cut my full membership, which included spinning class and other classes, as I was not intending to use those, and it saved me a lot of money.

It felt amazing to be so focused again on my personal goal and I was reminded of memorable moments from my early career, which had influenced my life, and they were guiding me again in this moment of need.

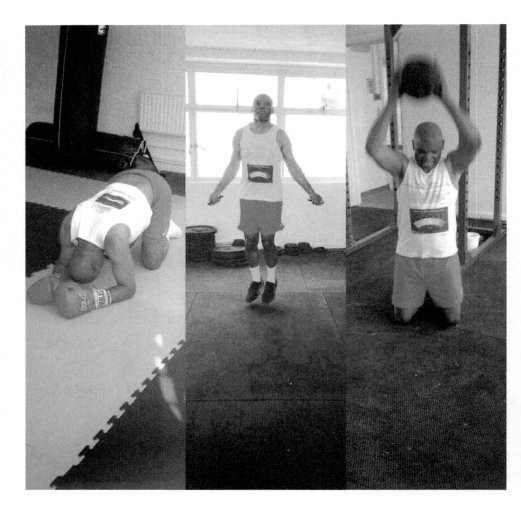

Flashback 4:
My network marketing experience when I was a young adult trying to earn a living in London

I was on my way home on a warm Friday afternoon in the summer from The Savoy Hotel to Covent Garden tube station when a young man, who later became my sponsor, approached me and asked if I wanted to earn some extra money. Well, of course, as a young man, this sounded good, and after a short conversation, I said yes, so he gave me details of a meeting on the Monday evening. I attended the meeting and was surprise to see the room packed with people. We were shown a business plan and told about the potential of working independently, with possible travel, extra income and new products to sample. What really attracted me was that we would get paid for using the products. Because I was already a professional chef, I really liked it when they spoke about nutrition and wellness and I signed up that same night. As I became more involved and studied the products, I learnt the importance of supplements in my diet and I have been taking the Nutrilite products ever since those early days of my career.

It was a significant experience for me at a young age because it helped me develop several critical life skills. I learnt more about nutrition and health, I was part of a community of like-minded people, and I had support within this association.

They gave us personal mentoring and skills development in areas including: communicating with customers; and effective sales and marketing. Network marketing also provided us with tapes, mentoring books and CDs of successful people for us to listen to and learn from. These became a great foundation for my development and helped me hugely in future challenges in my life.

At the start of 2016, when I reset my focus and was determined to achieve my weight lose and blood glucose reduction goal, I began doing more detailed research on dietary food. I realised I had to cut out all carbohydrates from my list of food to eat and I took it literally, especially the starchy ones including: rice; potato; and pasta, which had all been my regular consumption. I went to the supermarket and looked at every package, reading all the labels, to find products without carbohydrates. To my surprise, it was hard to find products without carbohydrates.

I made the decision to only eat the food I like for my diet that would be beneficial. This meant that I used red onions when frying, coconut oil, olive oil or nutty oil. I loved making stir-fries with sweetcorn, peppers, kale, spinach, grilled chicken, salmon or cod. This is an example of my basic food. I simply cooked and combined any of the food from my list, as detailed in Chapter 5: Crossing the Threshold and Committing to Change: going cold turkey.

I remember one experience that had an affect on my thinking at this time. One evening I was watching a TV programme about an overweight family who were unaware of the illnesses they might have if they continued doing what they were doing. They had a doctor with them helping them to understand the implications of what they were eating and how this was going to affect their lives negatively in the future. They put a healthy plan of action together, including blood tests, exercise, nutrition and an analyse of the food they were eating. When the blood test came back, the husband was diagnosed with type 2 diabetes and other symptoms, and he was prescribed a selection of medicines. The family was shocked and it was a dark emotional moment for them all. I remember the wife saying with tears in her eyes, 'I can't believe it. We always thought we were eating healthly.'

It was difficult for this family to change their established habits and it was so serious that the doctor working with them suggested they had a 24-hour fast with no food. The husband was not losing weight and the doctor explained the benefits of fasting and how it can help radically. That put a light on in my head, and I said to myself, 'I am going to take fasting more seriously, starting from tomorrow and only drink water.' I had fasted before, as I have mentioned earlier, but only before having a blood test and only for 12-15 hours, when I was asleep most of the time anyway.

There were periods of time, when working as a chef, you went five to six hour periods without food anyway, with only a tea, coffee or cigarette break. In some restaurant establishments, they did not feed you and the chefs bought their food in or went to the shops to buy lunch. In the early days of going to the gym, I did not have anything to eat. When I knew I was going to the gym, I drank water only and this soon became a regular routine. I was conscious of what I was doing and when I felt like eating, I drank water instead. Subconsciously, I was fasting. I had it in my mind if I don't eat food, my sugar level will be low.

The next morning, I had porridge with blueberries and 80% dark chocolate before I started my fast for the rest of that day. I was sitting in my car eating the porridge thinking, 'Am I doing the right thing by fasting for 24 hours?' I was thinking about getting hungry and wanting something nice to eat and thoughts of food were playing around in my head. I took my last spoonful of porridge and as I licked the spoon, it was right on 9am. I got into the motion of the day and when it reached the time when I usually had a break from working and had something to eat, my stomach rumbled but my mind said no! I looked at my water bottle and had a drink. Every time I had that hunger reminder, I drank more water. I was pre-occupied throughout the day, which made it easier. It was a full-on challenging day and by the evening I still had the hunger pains and could not wait to go to bed to forget about it.

The next morning, I woke up at 8am and felt really hungry but my fast was to end at 9am and I had to wait before I allowed myself any breakfast! In the mornings, I am usually up early and on the telephone or computer getting busy. I usually take my daughter to netball on a Saturday at about 9.15am and at 9am on that particular morning, when my 24-hour fast ended, it was a anti-climax. I thought I would dive into the fridge, bread bin or get something to eat, but I actually did not feel like it. I decided to take Jasmine to netball and have something when I got back. I had water in the car and I drank that. When I came home about 10am, 25 hours now into my fast, I simply drank more water.

It is a good time to catch up with my wife on Saturday mornings when she was not working in London, and usually we are deep in conversation. I did not think about eating and I said to myself, 'I'm going to do a 26-hour fast,' and I achieved that goal.

It was a challenge, but after all the anxiety, I did not really feel hungry because the water was efficient.

I remember my wife was watching a weight loss programme on television and I was on the other side of the room. They mentioned the celebrities who were on a weight loss diet drinking cayenne pepper water. I was in the kitchen in seconds and adding cayenne pepper to my water bottle. I made a jug of it for the next morning, mixing it with the fresh lemon juice in my recipe already. However, when I tasted it, I was not ready for the spiciness and it made me cough! But if it was going to work, I had to drink it, so I did!

One of the most exciting times for me was when I was in the gym on the cross trainer and I felt the cayenne pepper kick in and make me sweat more. This experience was motivating and it helped me to go faster and burn more.

I continued in my five fast track routine, focusing my attention on my: mindset; food; flavonoids; fasting; and exercise. But then I added a new experience to my recipe for recovery and I attended the diabetes course offered by the NHS.

Being a chef and interested in food and nutrition, I went to all of the four sessions of the diabetes course that I was offered in January 2016. In particular, I wanted to see if they would mention flavonoids in any of these sessions, but of the four I attended, these were never mentioned once! Each session was only two hours long.

NHS Record of the diabetes courses Lyndon attended in January 2016

Date	Title	Topic
13 January	Session One: Starting Life with Diabetes	An overview of the issues surrounding type 2 diabetes
16 January	Session Two: Diet and You	The dietary principles of living with diabetes, led by a dietician
20 January	Session Three: Targets and Terminology	Led by a physiotherapist to explain the benefits of activity and taking control of your diabetes
27 January	Session Four: Foot Care and Medication	Led by a podiatrist to discuss good foot ache and a specialist nurse to discuss medication

When I attended my first session, it was a time of anticipation and quite an exciting time for me, waiting for the information to help me get to the next level. This was especially the case for me because I had waited for two and half months for this course, from my diagnosis in October 2015 to January 2016.

I remember the first day clearly, as I walked in and took a seat quietly. There was an air of stillness in the room with quiet conversations going on in small groups. There was a table in the middle of the classroom with artificial food items in the centre. For example: egg; macaroni; potato; baked beans; cheese; and bacon.

There was a tick sign at one end of the table and a cross sign at the other end of the table. We were asked to put the foods into the tick area or the cross area. This was to determine what foods we were able to eat or not able to eat as diabetics. This got the people in the class out of their seats and participating. The conversation was good about what foods we can eat or not; it was, yes, no or maybe answers and everyone joined in! Some people were sure and others were not. We finally finished and sat down and we were given booklets about food. The nutritionist continued with the session covering good foods and the foods we should avoid, for example, carbohydrates, GI foods and proteins.

They said the course is for preventative measures and care. We had a question and answer session on that day, they gave out cards with questions written on them and we had to answer right or wrong. In the class, there were middle-aged people upwards of all types of sizes, even slim people who you might think could not have diabetes.

On the first session, we had to go round and make introductions, giving our names and saying when and how long ago we had been diagnosed. That was good because it broke the ice as we shared our experiences one by one of being new or recently diagnosed. Several people were coming back for rejuvenation of information and to be reminded.

The course included lots of information about insulin, the pancreas and glucose, and what helps the food turn into glucose, such as carbohydrates. She also explained the differences between type 1 and type 2 diabetes. They talked about weight gathered around the waist and she gave an example of the pear and apple shape. This related to me because I was losing most of my weight around my waistline. She explained how important exercise was. As we got into the questions, the session became quite heated. The questions came flooding in and people were shaking their heads, saying they were confused because the information we were getting from the dietician was not the same as the research we were all doing on the internet.

She explained about portion sizes and the importance of controlling how much we ate of each food according to its sugar content. One large gentleman said that what she was giving us as a recommendation was not a portion. He repeated it several times saying it would not fill him up. We all made helpful suggestions to him, including that maybe he could have a couple of glasses of water before eating his meal. He was very unhappy and did not respond, even though we were talking about food in our diet and the role it plays.

Through my research and from what my cousin Ken had told me, I knew how important the pancreas is as an organ to produce insulin. Yet there was no mention in this first diabetes course of food to help the pancreas, such as flavonoids. They told us that once we were on Metformin, we would always be on it. Nobody had been suggested to come off Metformin from their dietician, even though their HbA1c level had reduced. I mentioned blueberries and she said all berries are good, and did not expand on this or what their benefits are. I felt as if I could have added more information to seriously help the other people in the room. To my way of thinking, there seemed to be so much good information that we were not being given. I was confused about this.

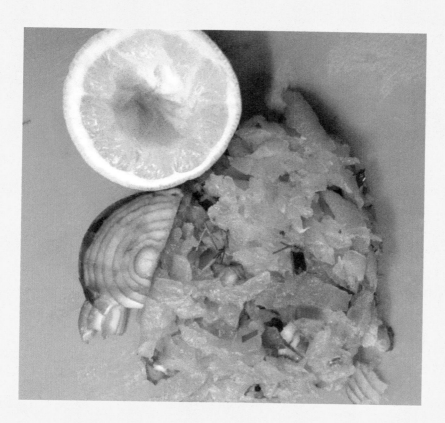

Lyndon's eyes

OD
Field: CENTRAL
Date: 20-09-2016 04:24 PM
Pupil size 4.3mm

OS
Field: CENTRAL
Date: 20-09-2016 04:25 PM
Pupil size 4.1mm

PATIENT'S NOTES:

EXAM'S NOTES: EXAM'S NOTES:

Lyndon's diabetic eye screening results: one of the symptoms of type 2 diabetes is blurred vision. It is also the most common cause of blindness in working-age diabetics. This specific eye screen result shows that Lyndon had no retina damage and the doctor told him how good this was. Lyndon had been taking vitamin supplements, including: Lutein and Zeaxanthin; Bilberry; and Beta-carotene supplements, on a regular basis for many years, before being diagnosed. Lyndon also ate fresh blueberries as his fruit snack and believes these made a difference for him.

Chapter 10

Physical Awareness: take care of your eyes and your feet

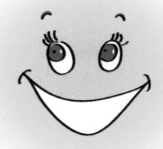

Eye Care

One of my early diabetic memories was of a warm sunny morning, when I not looking forwards to the one-mile walk from home to the hospital where I was booked in for an eye test. But we had no car that day and my daughters were coming to keep me company as far as the hospital and then they had something else to do in town. As I walked with Jasmine and Nadia, it was at a quick pace that I was not used to because that journey was usually taken by car and normally takes five minutes, without traffic.

As we walked, I felt myself starting to panting and breathe heavily and my heart beating faster and I said, 'You girls really walk fast.'

They both giggled simultaneously and said this was their normal pace. I shook my head, glared into the sky as the sun shone bright and thought I'll need those sunglasses I was advised to bring! I remembered my cousin telling me that he had his dark glasses but didn't need them as it was a dull day. My thoughts went back to where I was going, anticipating arriving at the automatic doors to see the reception desk, where someone normally told me where to go.

But when I arrived, no one was there and I was staring at the signs to see which direction to go. I finally saw the right stairs with the cold metal rails and I went to the second floor to the waiting area. A lady dressed in a nurse outfit asked me if I was there for an eye test and when I said yes, she asked my name and told me to sit down.

As I walked towards a chair, looking for a comfortable spot to have my own little space, I saw a worn-out wooden box with leaflets on top. My curiosity got the best of me and I walked across the room to have a look. There were lots of different subject leaflets but the interesting one was about eye care. I flicked through the pages and to my surprise one of them mentioned the supplements Lutein and Zeaxanthin. I searched deep into my thoughts to recall where I had seen these words before. Then I remembered I was taking these supplements already. It was a feeling of relief because maybe I was using the right supplements for one of the ailments that may cause my eyes to be damaged by the diabetes.

There were a couple more leaflets on the shelf and I took those as well. As I sat back down in my seat with a handful of leaflets, I started to flick through them, but in my mind, I was thinking about the stinging sensation I would get when the eye drops go into my eyes. When the nurse called me, I walked around to a small table and chair and made myself comfortable. She asked me if I had my sunglasses with me and I responded that I did. She reminded me about the stinging sensation I was about to experience and then she asked me to put to my head back. When I leaned back, I saw this person lean over me and I watched this small tube of liquid drop into my eye. I squinted as it hit my eye and felt a sharp sting. It wasn't as bad as I had thought it would be. But then the same procedure happened again with the other eye. When that was finished, I went back to my seat and had to sit quietly for about 15 minutes with the tingling feeling in my eyes. Soon it was my turn to go to be tested and I walked into the dimly lit room where the optician was sitting.

There was a large machine in front of where I had to sit down and the optician asked me to put my chin on the machine. He asked me to look into the lens with my left eye and tell him when I saw the red spot. I said, 'I can't see a red spot.' He said me to look again and I said, 'I still can't see a red spot.' He asked me to try with the other eye and I moved away from machine for a second, blinking to refocus my eyes before putting my chin back on the machine. I looked into the lens again, and by some miracle I saw the red spot in the centre of the lens.

He told me to follow the green light with my eyes. It was at the bottom of the lens, and as he clicked the machine, my eye followed the green light. This took place with both eyes separately and then he took photos of my eyes. When the light flashed, it was temporarily blinding and my eyes were blurry. When that was done, he showed me the pictures of the blood vessels at the back of my eyes and told me the great news that I had no damage and my eyes were in good shape. As we were finishing off, I was waiting to be given some eye care advice but he said nothing and so I plucked up the courage and asked him what I could do to maintain this.

He simply told me to take supplements, so I mentioned to him about eating kale and asked him what he thought. But his response was pretty unhelpful, I thought. He simply said, 'Oh yeah, it's a good thing to have any leafy greens in your diet.' I was disappointed because he was the expert and I thought he should be telling me this advice, rather than me having to ask the questions of him!

As we finished our conversation, we walked into the corridor, past the leaflets on the shelves, and I thought maybe he would direct me in their direction for more eye care information, but we walked straight past them.

We said goodbye and I left, walking back to the concrete stairs. As I left the hospital, it seemed much busier but I knew I was meant to put the sunglasses on, and yet I was very aware of all the people around me. Would they be watching me and wondering why I was wearing these sunglasses inside?

Diabetes can affect your eyes because it is part of a group classified as retinal vascular disorders. In a worst case scenario, diabetes, if untreated, can cause blindness. It is therefore essential to look after your eyes if you are diagnosed and actually before that by taking precautionary steps to prevent any visual loss. Out of the

3.5 million diabetic patients in the UK, each person has a 10 to 20 per cent chance of losing their eyesight.

Crucially, diabetes, when detected at an early stage, can be managed effectively and be prevented from causing lasting complications. Insulin-dependent diabetes (IDD), known as type 1, can develop between 10 and 20 years of age generally, although some elderly people may be classified as IDD. Type 2 diabetes is also known as a non-insulin-dependent diabetes (NIDD), but most frequently when patients are between the age of 50 and 70 years old.

The first signs of diabetes affecting your eyes can be found in the retina, which is the light sensitive most inner layer of the eye. The retina is the photosensitive part of the eye, which collects images and sends them to the brain for interpretation through the optic nerve. If the retina is damaged, it pixels the light sensitive cells and affects the image quality. The vision is impaired. Once you have the signs of damage to your retina, it is called Diabetic Retinopathy (DR). This is prevalent in 40% of IDDs and 20% of NIDDs.

The eye can be explained in the same way as a camera. A traditional film in a vintage camera is the same as the retina and if the film is damaged, the image produced will be of lower quality. The same applies to the retina. Regardless of how well the lens is or how well the refraction of the eye is, if the retina is damaged the vision is hard to improve with lenses. Blood vessels irrigate the retina and if you are a diabetic, those blood vessels can become weak and cause vascular changes. As a patient, you might not be aware of this damage but if you leave it untreated, it can be very serious indeed.

This will cause the (DR) to be proliferative. This means new blood vessels will grow and be proliferate on the optic nerve head. This process is called Neovascularization. What is amazing throughout this process, is that patients are not aware of the changes happening to their eyes.

However, this can be treated by laser, to prevent recurrent haemorrhage.

Risk factors which contribute to eye damage include the following:

- duration of the condition;
- poor diabetic control;
- hypertension;
- recent cataract surgery;
- pregnancy;
- alcohol abuse; and
- smoking.

Prevention is better and cheaper than cure.

A routine eye test should be carried out every two years, if you suspect diabetes is a problem. Mention this to your optometrist who will refer you to your doctor and include registration at your nearest hospital for an annual diabetic retinal screening. Thankfully, all these contingencies are supported by the National Health Service in the UK. It is also important to be aware of your family history because eye problems are hereditary and the most important message as a diabetic is for you to always keep up to date with regular check-ups. Complications can be discovered quickly and managed effectively.

LYNDON'S CHOICE OF FOODS TO HELP WITH EYE CARE

Food	Goodness
Dragon fruit	Vitamin C to protect and nourish the cornea
Kiwano	Vitamin A and Beta-carotene to protect the surface of the eye
Kale and all leafy green vegetables	Range of vitamins
Lutein and Zeaxanthin	Blood vessel care
Buddha's head	Vitamin C
Mangosteen	Multiple vitamin B complex
Jack fruit	Vitamin C
Custard apple	Vitamins C and B with potassium
Rambuton	Vitamin B and bioflavonoids
Linseed (oil and ground meal)	Omega 3 good fats

Durwin Banks, owner and farmer at the British Linseed Farm in Sussex, UK provided Lyndon with the following contribution.

What can a plant that would have been part of the medicine chest belonging to Hippocrates do to help with diabetic problems? Well, this plant can be a fundamental dietary staple helping to stabilise blood sugar levels and provide fats that are required for the proper functioning of the pancreas. So what is this plant? The answer is linseed, often called flaxseed by the Americans; its Latin name *Linum usitatissimum*, means 'most useful'. Linseed is increasingly being called a superfood and there are good reasons for this. One of them is the help it can give in supporting people with diabetes or likely to move towards having a diabetic condition.

Ground linseed meal is low on the Glycaemic index scale, referred to as GI. It is high in both soluble and insoluble fibre, which helps to slow the digestion and keep blood sugars more balanced. Linseed can do all this as part of your everyday food intake and it is gluten-free. Linseed contains useful amounts of iron magnesium, zinc and the important omega essential fatty acids.

Freshly ground linseed meal should be kept in the fridge ready to incorporate into everyday food. It can be stirred into porridge or added to smoothies; green vegetable are preferred to fruit types. Linseed itself tastes quite sweet but has no sugar and, mixed with porridge or yogurt for breakfast, can help reduce cravings during the mornings, it is also possible to make comforting snacks without being naughty.

Linseed meal supports your good gut bacteria and helps remove bad things as well. That's something Hippocrates was really interested in. He also promoted cider vinegar; the gut is the feeder of the whole body. It must be good to take more notice of some ancient wisdom. The Linseed Farm is sure that food is the best medicine, and linseed is one of the best.

To move on to the fatty acids, we need to have a balance of omega 3 and omega 6 of 1 to 1. Our food world has been overwhelmed with the omega 6 and the balance can be out by huge amounts 10/15/20, even 25%. No labels help you to eat the right balance so important for us stone-age people. The consequence of the imbalance is inflammation. Why? Omega 3 always produces anti-inflammatory hormones and omega 6 produces pro-inflammatory hormones. All the bodies systems need the right balance of fats to work at optimum efficiency and nowhere is this more important than for pancreatic function.

Think about it like this; as ancient people, we ran around and hunted and collected fruit, nuts and seeds. Our pancreas was fed with the best balance of fats to do its job, which is exactly the same job it does now. The difference is in the sugar intake. All the time, sugar and carbohydrates were in a reasonable balance, all was well and the mechanisms to keep your blood sugar levels regulated worked properly.

Move forward to our present day, and you find the wrong balance of fats ensuring the pancreas is not fed properly with far too many sugary and empty carbohydrates piled into our system.

You are asking a stone-age organ perfectly designed to keep us healthy with the correct care to do a job it is unable to perform for long periods of time and the result is diabetes.

Diabetes interferes with the healing processes of the body. It affects the eyes and results in amputations of legs or feet unable to heal themselves. Let me paint a picture for you. Those ancient people we have spoken about, they were hunter and gatherers and had innate knowledge of what to eat. When you see animals killed on the road, you will also see birds starting to peck at the eyes first and this is what we did in those ancient times, but why? The eyes contain lots of omega 3 fat as, of course, does the brain, and we ate that first as well.

This small insight makes us realise how important it is to supply our eyes with the right balance of fats. We, at the Linseed Farm, are hearing from more of our customers that their eye consultants and doctors are recommending linseed oil in general, but particularly for dry eyes. As the omega fats are so important, this is a heartening development and feedback is that linseed oil is helpful for eyes and, of course, you get extra good side effects as well.

Making simple changes and including linseed in your life will soon help you and eventually save huge sums of money spent to relieve the symptoms of a totally food-related disease.

It is estimated that the direct medical costs and the social costs may be as high as 50 billion pounds per year.

In my mind as a farmer, all this money is available for a better food system so we have plenty of money for good food, but we are giving it to the wrong people. My advice is to love linseed, and include more in your life. You will see more lovely blue fields in the countryside, and that will make everyone happy.

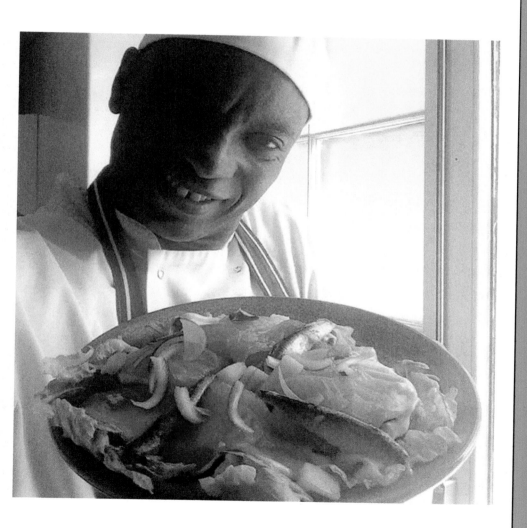

Foot care

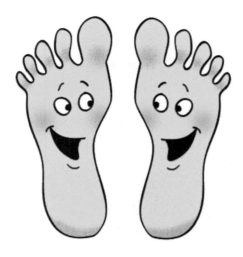

Being a chef, I need to look after my feet because I am standing on them all day in the kitchen and I very rarely sit down. For me, the most important thing I have done to look after my feet is to go for a regular pedicure, where my feet are massaged and nourished with moisturising cream, as well as having the nails properly cut and the dead skin removed. Doing this has really paid off for me and when my dietician asked to check my feet, she was surprised how healthy they were.

The doctors will recommend you go to see a podiatrist, which is the NHS process for foot care, but actually I have never had to do this because I had an established foot care regime already set up for myself and I have simply continued to visit my pedicurist because it works for me.

Lyndon's Seven Tips for Happy Feet

1. Understand the risks – understand what it means for your feet in particular as a diabetic. Go on all the NHS courses offered and research as much as you can and learn, learn, learn. Apply your new knowledge to look after yourself better.

2. Check your feet every day – look for any signs of redness, skin damage, bleeding and pain, and if in any doubt, go and see your doctor. Avoid using corn plasters and blades, because these can damage the skin. Also exercise your toes when you are checking your feet – wriggle them up and down and squeeze them in and out to give the circulation a boost.

3. Protect any problems with your feet – if you experience broken skins problems, keep them protected using dry sterile dressings. Check after two days that the sore is healing and if not, go and see your doctor.

4. Be aware of any loss of sensation in your feet – when you experience any changes to the feelings in your feet or you become aware of a tingling or numbness or regular feeling of pins and needles, go and see your doctor.

5. Wear properly fitting shoes and socks – be comfortable in your shoes and socks, and always buy shoes with adjustable fastenings so you can undo them easily and give your feet a rest. Change your socks or hosiery daily to maintain cleanliness.

6. Give your feet an MOT and have a regular pedicure – keep your toes clean and healthy and your toenails clean and well-trimmed. Have a regular foot massage and apply moisturiser to your feet daily to keep the skin in good condition, but not in-between the toes.

7. Keep up your glucose control – foot problems can be controlled with good glucose control and good, regular foot care. Remember, it is critically important that you keep the circulation active and the nerves and blood vessels healthy in your feet as a diabetic. After all, you use them every single day of your life, especially if you are a chef like me and you are standing up all day and moving around.

Chapter 11

Mastery of the Problem: success and elation!

The realisation that it was possible to actually achieve my goal grew gradually within my heart and kept me on track and totally motivated to win through. I attended regular blood glucose tests and slowly the numbers went down and down, and the knowledge that I was beating this condition called diabetes grew inside me and mainlined my dedicated mindset. In December 2015, my HbA1c level was down to 60 from 77. My goal was to reach the 50s at least, although the normal level of 42 would be even better, if I could really make it happen! When my dietician told me my level was down to 60, she said she had never had a patient who had done so well. Although this made me very happy and it silently spurned me on to keep reducing these levels, she never asked what I have been doing to be so successful nor considered sharing this information with anyone else!

My next blood test was booked for February 2016 and these results were becoming incredibly important for me. On the day of receiving those results, my body was in cold shivers of anticipation. As I entered the surgery, there was a queue and I felt like jumping the queue to know what my results were. I heard my voice quivering when I said to the receptionist I had come for my blood test results. She looked at her computer and she said it was

41 HbA1c. I looked at her in disbelief and asked her to confirm what she has just said. I could not believe what I was hearing. 'Are you sure?' I asked quietly. She repeated it and I was stunned, numbed, lips shivering as I slowly realised I had reversed my diabetes. I had controlled my diabetes. I had cured my diabetes. My words were being jumbled around in my head and my emotions were dancing all over the place inside me. I was fighting back the tears and clutching my fists as I asked the disinterested receptionist, 'Can I have a printout please?' She gave me the piece of paper with no understanding of what this meant to me, to my life, my family and all my friends at home and at work. I managed to say, 'Thank you,' with joy beginning to show up in my voice, my face, my emotions starting to come to the surface!

As I left the surgery, I did not even realise there was a queue behind me as I walked out with a bounce in my stride, then my emotions took over and the tears of relief and success ran down my cheeks. I was so the overwhelmed with joy, I could not call anybody straight away. I would not have been able to speak, not even to my wife. I kept thinking to myself, 'Below 42HbA1c is normal,' and I decided to book another blood test – just to be sure – because for the next four weeks, I needed to prove to myself that I was in control of this to confirm that I had achieved my goal. On the 29th February 2016, my next blood test confirmed my HbA1c level was 39 mmol/mol. I called my cousin Ken and I told him the wonderful news. He said, 'You cracked it, cousin. You did it. You cured it, well done!'

The moment I realised that I had actually succeeded in my quest to lose weight and reduce my blood glucose level to the normal, non-diabetic level, was a huge turning point in my life.

I had achieved an incredible goal, I had reversed, controlled, cured my diabetes! Wow, this was an extraordinary feeling!

My weight was down from 85/86 kilo to 76/77 kilo. I had changed my body shape, my face was thinner, my six-pack was showing and I felt great with all I had achieved! The remarkable thing that happened was I did not go the gym for two weeks, but I continued to lost weight and I was able to maintain it as I went back to eating in moderation the same foods I had been eating pre-diagnosis! I could only put it down to my daily lemon and cayenne pepper water because this was my regular drink. Also, I was drinking herb teas, either lemon and ginger or peppermint tea. I was going to the gym three times a week for two-hour sessions and I was eating carefully with a focus on my list of healthy food. I continue to drink my healthy cocktail with water and I know it is a combination of all these elements that make me feel and look so much better.

When I began realising what I had achieved, I started to talk about it to other people to spread the word to more people all over the world, and slowly the idea of writing this book began to take shape in my mind.

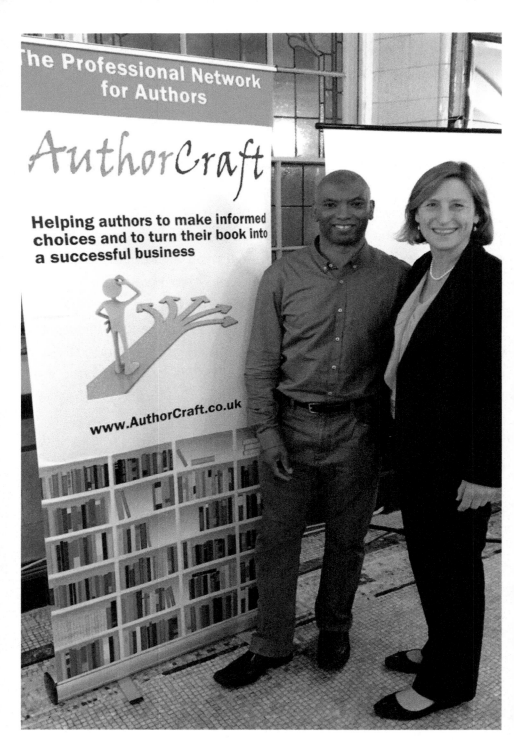

Lyndon with his Book Coach and Editor, Wendy Yorke

Final Flashback:

It was an eventful October 2015

I have a friend called Darren who had written a wonderful children's book, and when I told him about Ken and our idea or writing a book, he suggested we come to an AuthorCraft event. AuthorCraft is the Professional International Network for Authors, where authors meet and share their stories about their writing and book publishing journeys. They also help and support each other and it is run by a caring community of experts who provide professional advice from speakers in the industry. Attending an AuthorCraft event was an opportunity to meet people with similar stories to tell through their books and to learn new skills about writing and having a book published, as well as making connections with the experts to help authors to build businesses around their books.

That 24 November 2015 was a highly significant day for me because it was the day I learnt I had reversed my HbA1c level from 92mmol/mol to 77mmol/mol. I was incredibly excited and motivated and it was also the day I was meeting Ken to go to the AuthorCraft event together in the evening. I was dying to tell Ken my news and the day dragged along, but when I finally saw him and told him my results, he said, 'It's great what you have done and without medication, that is amazing.'

We went to the AuthorCraft event at the Institute of Directors, London and at the registration table, it was all smiles with an air of excitement. Darren was there to greet us and I introduced him to Ken. I could feel Darren's energy because he wanted us to meet Chris Day, the event founder and organiser. When we eventually met Chris and told him why we were there, he welcomed us openly and told us to enjoy the event and we would talk again. How right he was – because we have been talking ever since that first meeting, nearly every month at least!

I wanted to sit in the front row but the seats were taken, so I settled for the second row and Ken sat in the fourth or fifth row and I thought it must have been his comfort zone. But as I settled in my seat, I looked around and heard behind me a lot of conversations going on. I made eye contact with Ken and beckoned him to come and sit with beside and he came willingly. My thoughts were only to find out how to help Ken to write his book and tell his story by learning who was the best person for him to talk to. But as the evening went on, I became more and more excited, learning about the process of writing, editing and publishing.

During the break, I met a lady who had written about four books. My question to her was, 'Why do you write and where do you get the inspiration from?' She told me she enjoyed writing, but said clearly it was not for the money. Another person said to me they wrote books because they wanted to share their life story. This must have planted a subconscious seed in my head. The speakers at that event were brilliant. They included: Chris Day, the AuthorCraft orgainser and director of Filament Publishing; Helena Holrick, author and business coach; Carl Rosier-Jones, an author who was launching his book, *The Caveman Principles*, at the event; Janey Lee Grace, an author and media personality, also launching her new book at the event, *YOU are the BRAND*, and Wendy Yorke, author, editor and book coach, who spoke about 'Helping you be the best you can be.' What they all said really connected with me but it was Wendy who engaged my attention and resonated with me. It was only a few months later she became my book writing coach and editor.

Something happened that evening that made me realise maybe I had a story to tell too. Ken had reversed his type 1 diabetes and I was reversing my type 2. Together, we had a helpful story to tell other people that could help billions of sufferers all around the world. Two related stories with the same outcome - reversed diabetics.

I thought back to what Ken had said about reversing my diabetes without medication in such a short period of time. My dietician had also said she could not believe it and had never heard before of a patient who had done this. I went home thinking I could write a book to tell my story and I could help other people to achieve the same result that I had accomplished.

I thought about all the things that had happened to me since being diagnosed with type 2 diabetes; my emotions, my fears, my decisions and all the changes I had made in my life and now the amazing achievements. I thought too of my family, my work, my friends, how and who do I thank for all their support and help and guidance, and how could I share this with them all and with other people too. But I felt daunted by this idea at the same time, who might be able to help me with this task and at that stage I really did not know!

The next day, I researched books about how to reverse diabetes and I could not find one definitive person who said they had reversed their diabetes. I called my friend Nick, who was into yoga and healthy eating and is very knowledgeable about natural food. He mentioned a book by a doctor and I followed up this lead and

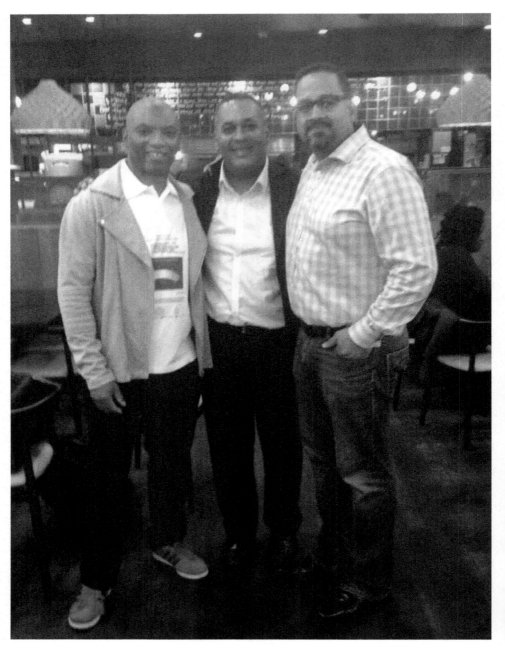

Lyndon with Richard Icare (centre) and Sherwyn Singh, who have supported him every step of his journey.

did some more research of his methods. But I was not happy enough within myself about the stories I was finding because no one had written about how it was actually possible to reverse, control and ultimately cure type 2 diabetes and I had just achieved this! So I decided to call Darren and thank him for the AuthorCraft evening, but also to inform him that I wanted to tell my story and to write this book.

Chapter 12
Pre-Diabetes Check List and Action Plan:

plus Lyndon's Five Fast Track Recipe to reversing, controlling and curing type 2 diabetes

Pre–Diabetes Check List

When you suspect you are pre-diabetic but you have not yet been tested nor had it confirmed, you can change your diet immediately. Use the food and drinks listed in Chapter 5: Crossing the Threshold and Committing to Change: going cold turkey.

Pre-Diabetics Action Plan
Before your HbA1c test to find out if you are diabetic or not, follow the Action Plan below which worked to reduce Lyndon's levels. If you can reduce your levels before your test, you can avoid being diagnosed as a diabetic.

Think about what you would like to have hear from your doctor or dietician after being diagnosed as a diabetic.

This is the information that would have helped Lyndon through his recovery. He worked it out for himself through his dedicated mindset and focused approach.

- Cut out as much carbohydrates as possible in your food intake.
- Base all your meals around flavonoids.
- Ensure all your food consist of blood glucose reducing ingredients.
- Exercise and lose weight according to your BMI (Body Mass Index).
- Seek professional advice and support to monitor your progress.
- Reduce your sugar intake from food and drinks.
- Have a strong mindset and belief you can do it.
- Be disciplined and focused.
- Ensure you have supportive people around you.
- Drink lemon water and plenty of water all the way through your day, every day.

Lyndon's Five Fast Track Recipe to Reversing, Controlling and Curing Type 2 Diabetes

1. Mindset

"A person without a goal has nothing to aim for."

Mental focus is allowing the self-talk to set your mind on the direction toward the goals that you know is right for you. It is affirming what you specifically want. This is a personal choice, for example, a weight loss goal, or a HbA1c level reduction goal.

2. Food

Food is the key to keeping your blood sugar levels down. My daily okra and lemon water drink was the key element that worked for me, avoiding the sweet, hot and cold fizzy drinks, and knowing what to do instead.

3. Flavonoids

Flavonoids are the food that heal and nourish the pancreas. Keeping it nourished helps to produce insulin.

4. Fasting

This is probably the most difficult ingredient of my diabetes cure recipe because as human beings, we always want to eat solid food when that hunger pain kicks in. However, be strong and kick it out with water or your special formulated drink. Especially in the mornings, it is a good test to only drink water for a couple of hours and you can increase the time you last slowly and gradually building it up. There are plenty of health benefits well documented from responsible and controlled fasting for short periods only.

5. Exercise

Who really likes to exercise? The reason the majority of us are where we are is because of a lack of exercise! We simply have to accept that our bodies need physical exercise. For me, it was finding what I enjoyed the most and what fitted into my work and home routine. And you can do the same, be it at home, in the gym, or whatever suits you.

I wish you success on your journey, and please keep me informed of your progress.

I believe in you:
#SelfCuredDiabeticNaturally

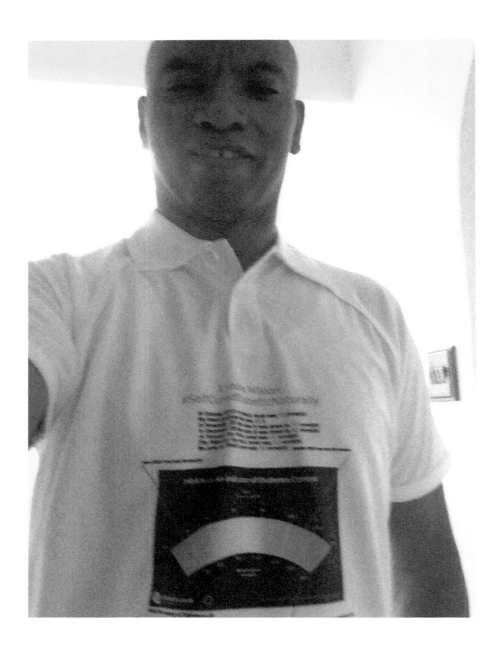

Share your story with me on Twitter, Facebook and my
website at www.lyndonwissart.com

APPENDIX

Type 2 diabetes can be cured through weight loss, Newcastle University finds

Millions of people suffering from Type 2 diabetes could be cured of the disease if they just lost weight, a new study suggests.

Scientists at Newcastle University have shown the disease is caused by fat accumulating in the pancreas and losing less than one gram from the organ can reverse the life-limiting illness and restore insulin production.

Type 2 diabetes affects 3.3 million people in England and Wales and, until now, was thought to be chronic. It can lead to blindness, stroke, kidney failure and limb amputation.

"For people with type 2 diabetes, losing weight allows them to drain excess fat out of the pancreas and allows function to return to normal" Professor Roy Taylor, Newcastle University.

But now researchers at Newcastle have shown that the disease can be reversed, even in obese people who have had the condition for a long time.

18 obese people with type 2 diabetes who were given gastric band surgery and put on a restricted diet for eight weeks were cured of

their condition. During the trial the patients, aged between 25 and 65, lost an average of 2.2 stone, which was around 13 per cent of their body weight. Crucially, they also lost 0.6 grams of fat from their pancreas, allowing the organ to secrete normal levels of insulin.

The team is now planning a larger two year study involving 200 people with Glasgow University to check that the findings can be replicated and weight loss can be sustained for two years.

In the UK, 64 per cent of adults are classed as being overweight, meaning their body mass index (BMI) is greater than 25.

"For people with type 2 diabetes, losing weight allows them to drain excess fat out of the pancreas and allows function to return to normal," said Professor Roy Taylor, of Newcastle University who also works within the Newcastle Hospitals.

"So if you ask how much weight you need to lose to make your diabetes go away, the answer is one gram. But that gram needs to be fat from the pancreas. At present the only way we have to achieve this is by calorie restriction by any means, whether by diet or an operation.

"What is interesting is that regardless of your present body weight and how you lose weight, the critical factor in reversing your type 2 diabetes is losing that one gram of fat from the pancreas."

Source: The Telegragh, 1 December 2015

Oskar Minkowski

Lyndon researched the following information online, about Oskar Minkowski who discovered pancreatic diabetes, from the global diabetes community at www.diabetes.co.uk/research.html

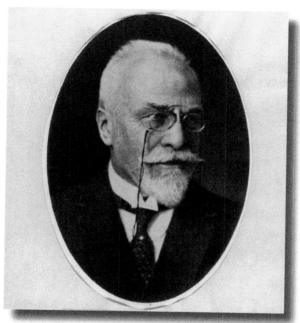

Oskar Minkowski is famous for his discovery of pancreatic diabetes and he was nominated for the Nobel Prize six times during his career. Minkowski studied at the University of Konigsberg, Austria before becoming a professor in Strasburg in 1888.

Minkowski discovered a library journal in which Joseph von Mering asserted that pancreatic enzymes were required to breakdown fatty acids in the gut. According to physiologist Claude Bernard, performing a pancreatectomy (surgical removal of the pancreas), which would be the best way of establishing this assertion, was impossible, but Minkowski proceeded to conduct the procedure in dogs.

Von Mering was Minkowski's assistant for the procedure and after Minkowski made the connection between polyuria and diabetes, he tested the urine of the animals for glucose. The high glucose levels marked the discovery of pancreatic diabetes.

Minkowski went on to chair the German Association of Internal Medicine and became one of Europe's leading dialectologists. Since 1966, the Minkowski Prize for outstanding contribution to the advancement of knowledge in the field of Diabetes Mellitus has been awarded by the European Association for the Study of Diabetes.

Lyndon researched online about spirulina and okra, from the global diabetes community at http://www.diabetes.co.uk/natural-therapies/okra.html

Lyndon researched the benefits of eating okra on the following website: http://www.healthline.com/health/diabetes/okra#

Lyndon researched the benefits of eating psyllium from the University of Maryland Medical Centre, website as follows: http://umm.edu/health/medical/altmed/supplement/psyllium

Lyndon researched a good site called 'Heal Naturally' which provides responsible healing information and can be accessed from the following website: http://www.realnatural.org/category/health/

Lyndon investigated the question 'Is olive leaf nature's answer to diabetes treatment?' from the 'Heal Naturally' link: http://www.realnatural.org/is-olive-leaf-natures-answer-to-diabetes-treatment/

Lyndon used the following website to research 'Why drinking lemon water is good for you?' at: https://healthunlocked.com/diabetesindia/posts/130246945/why-you-should-drink-lemon-water-in-the-morning

Lyndon also used the following websites to research the health benefits of cloves in his diet: https://www.organicfacts.net/health-benefits/herbs-and-spices/health-benefits-of-cloves.html

http://www.newsmax.com/Health/Headline/Mediterranean-diet-heart-disease-cancer-spices/2013/04/04/id/497912/

http://www.livestrong.com/article/477349-cinnamon-cloves-and-diabetes/

Support for Lyndon from around the world, from family and friends

'Lyndon, congratulations on your journey. I am very happy with what you've achieved and definitely it needs to be promoted, so other people can benefit from your story.'
Piotr

'Wow, Lyndon, this is amazing!! That is discipline. Well done, proud of you.'
Richard

'That is absolutely REMARKABLE!!! Well done you for being able to drop from the extremely high levels to normal ones so quickly! I hope it stays below 40 from now on and you will be OK!'
Dina

'Amazing, Lyndon! I am so pleased for you. You must feel fabulous.'
H

'Well done! Your journey to be drug free of diabetes will be an inspiration to others when they read your story. Keep up the good word! All the best.'
Chris

'Wow, Lyndon, you defy gravity! Well done!!! Start writing that book! One copy sold for sure already.'
Jo

'Oh my days, dat is blessed news, my brudda ...D u feel good?'
Bevan

'So happy to hear! Well done! Keep up. Take care.'
Anca

'Great news, very glad to hear that you are making such great progress.'
Jacques

'That is so great and exciting, Lyn. Perfect, my friend, I'm excited as well now.'
Nick

'That's amazing, mate, honestly incredible! Hopefully see you soon!'
Ed

'That's absolutely incredible! More than what you could have hoped for at the start and amazing for the project too. It's a sign, this has to be smashed!'
Obie

'That's brilliant, Lyndon!'
Anne-Marie

'Mate, that's amazing. Good for you, pal.'
Ross

'Great news. You must have been very strict to reduce it so much.'
Celia

'Fantastic news, well done.'
Peter

'Well done! You are champion.'
Slavo

'Wow, that's great news. It just shows what effect diet and exercise can have on your body. Very well done!'
Angela

'That's fantastic news about your bloods! Very impressive that it's just been lowered with diet and exercise.'
Liam

'Good for u, my friend.'
Sherena

'That's great news, Lyndon. I'm proud of your determination. The world needs to know about it.'
Martin

'That's great, congratulations.'
Marta

'No Meds Cured. Amazing with the 39 score. Crazy, how it's dramatically dropped.'
Leon

'Amazing! Your book is going to be an inspiration.'
Luke

'You have done brilliantly. Role model, I always believed in you.'
Karen

'You are amazing!'
Yvonne

'Great news for the day! Keep up the good work.'
Danielle

'Amazing, Lyndon. Taking charge. Like the title nice and simple.'
Darren

'Fantastic news, Lyndon! This is such a good result. It is possible to change your fortune. You've just proven it. Again! I'm proud of you.'
Sherwyn

'I am really happy for you because you deserve it! You are a wonderful friend, boss, colleague and, the most important, you are great as a human being! Good luck with all you want to do in your life!!'
Mihaela Andreica

'Brilliant! I look forward to hearing all the elements that contributed to your curing yourself of diabetes with no medication, no medication and no medication - that is the exciting part!! Good for you. Live long and strong!'
Lydia Keles

'Lyndon- you are an inspiration; I wish you continued good health for many years to come and look forward to reading your story.'
Dennis Daye

'Wow, well done, Lyndon. Let us know a bit more about it.'
Denilson Cerqueira

'Great stuff, Lyndon. Well done for turning something negative into something so positive.'
Angela Reid

'Lyndon, you are inspirational.'
Celia Clyne

Share your story with me on...

Twitter: @lwissart
Facebook: lwissart
my website: www.lyndonwissart.com

Lightning Source UK Ltd.
Milton Keynes UK
UKOW07f0159130117

292006UK00010B/51/P